MW00355834

MAKING PEACE WITH HERPES

A HOLISTIC GUIDE TO OVERCOMING THE STIGMA AND FREEING YOURSELF FROM OUTBREAKS

GREEN
SUN

CHRISTOPHER SCIPIO
HERBALIST — HOLISTIC VIRAL SPECIALIST

Making Peace With Herpes:
A Holistic Guide to Overcoming the Stigma and Freeing Yourself from
Outbreaks.

Copyright 2006-15 Christopher Scipio

All rights reserved. No part of this publication may be reproduced or
transmitted in any form, by any means electronic or mechanical including
photocopying, recording or any other information or retrieval system
without the written permission of Christopher Scipio, except in the case
of brief quotations that are part of articles or reviews.

Published by
Green Sun Press
5330 Snodgrass Road
Sechelt, BC, Canada, v0n 3a2
www.herpesbook.com

Cover design and page layout by Christopher Scipio
Photo of Christopher Scipio by Jamie Kowal

Printed in The USA

First Printing 2006
Second Printing 2009
Third Printing 2015
ISBN 0-9780780-3-9

For my mother,
my daughter,
and Ishil

How To Get This Book For Free?

If after reading this book you're interested
in having a phone consultation to ask questions,
get support and advice or wish to start
my holistic herpes treatment programme-
I will deduct the price of this book from
the cost of your phone consultation. Please either
write to me directy at christopher.scipio@gmail.
com or book your consultation through my site at
http://www.natropractica.com

Contents

Preface:

This isn't a book just about herpes. If you want to read a book that discusses the virus in depth from a scientific point of view but explained so that non-scientists can understand it, then I would recommend reading "The Truth About Herpes" by Dr. Stephen Sacks. This book doesn't acknowledge that there are effective natural treatments for herpes but I will forgive the late Dr. Sacks for his bias since he was a scientist. I will now admit to my own bias. I believe that Natural healing should be a first option rather than a therapy of last resort after drug-therapy has failed and loaded your body with toxins.

The simple truth is that unless you need to go to the emergency room or require surgery, you can treat most chronic illnesses just as well if not better with natural medicine, than you can with drug therapy. I also don't subscribe to the belief that natural medicine needs to be validated by a hostile scientific community that is motivated to discredit natural therapies in order to preserve their power and wealth. Natural medicine has been validated over and over again for thousands of years because it simply works. Common sense and intelligence are not recent developments in human history. Some people may believe their ancestors were clueless - I am not one of them.

Herbal medicine and holistic healing has survived for three hundred centuries because it works and produces results. I for one didn't wait for the scientists to begrudgingly admit to the medical benefit of garlic when I knew the Egyptian doctors had already validated it some 3500 years ago.

You will find no references to any clinical studies in this book. The knowledge I am sharing with you is knowledge I have acquired through treating my own herpes for 24 years and from being a working holistic herpes treatment specialist with a busy international practice that treats hundreds of herpes patients every year. I don't get my knowledge from second or third hand sources. I get to experience every day what works and doesn't work for people trying to manage their herpes holistically. I have also had the privilege of being guided in my work by some of the best herbalists, botanists, phycologists and mycologists in North America.

This is not a book just about herpes but is a book about living a holistically healthy life for those like myself who have a life-long herpes infection.

There is no cure for herpes and there isn't likely to be a cure in my lifetime or yours. When you read my chapter on the nature of the herpes virus you will see why the herpes virus is so challenging to cure. And to put things in perspective we cannot cure the common cold, or the flu, or chicken-pox, or almost any other viral infection. We still live in a society still very much afriad and ignorant of viruses. The medical community has not produced many effective anti-viral drugs as yet. In the near future there will be a vaccine to protect those uninfected with herpes from being infected, but as of today that isnt a reality.

The good news and the ironic news is that herpes is one of the easiest diseases to manage naturally. There is absolutely no need to take drug-therapy for herpes.

This book isn't just about how to have fewer outbreaks or how to stop having outbreaks; just doing that isn't enough to be healthy. This book is about holistically healing your herpes and living a healthy, happy and balanced life. Holistic health is about much more than making symptoms go away.

Every disease can be healed. Not every person will be healed.

Being healed is significantly different than being "cured".

You can be healed of herpes but you cannot be "cured". To be cured would mean that there is no more virus in your body. That isn't possible at the present; however you can be healed.

Healing is a return to balance, to equilibrium, to homeostasis, to a state of grace.

You can achieve all of this with the virus still in your body.

A great healer once told me that it was almost pointless to heal someone if they were not going to learn something in the process. Healing is about learning and growing; about becoming a better human being. You cannot be healed and expect to be the same person you were when you were diseased. You will have to change your ways, change your thinking, change your expectations, and change your beliefs.

You will need to stop your toxic habits and toxic thoughts. You will have to treat your body with more respect. Don't expect holistic healing to work if you are unwilling to give up your recreational drugs, or cigarettes or coffee or other bad habits that may be weakening your body's ability to heal.

There is an ocean of love and mercy around us at all times, ready, willing and able to assist in our healing. To receive your healing you can tune into this life-force anytime. The only thing keeping you apart from this ultimate healing is the illusion of separation.

To receive your healing, chant down your skepticism. To receive your healing let go of your attachment to your disease. To receive your healing dispel your notion of yourself as being a diseased person - and instead see yourself as a person who was once diseased and out of balance and is now progressing towards balance and health. See yourself as a person being healed. Claim your healing. It is your God/dess given right.

And last but not least. Get out of the way of your own healing. In all things in life, you are your own biggest obstacle.

If you think these are a bunch of New Age slogans, I have to tell you that you are mistaken. First of all I am not New Age; I come from a healing tradition that is very OldAge. Herbal Medicine has been the chief healing modality for human beings for at least 30,000 years and continues to be the main therapy for 70% of the world's population today. Compare that to the only 75 years of existence of modern western medicine; the Johnny-come-lately of the healing world. Holistic healing has been the way all cultures around the world have addressed health issues. Holistic healing is the best and only sustainable way of managing a lifelong herpes infection.

My Pitch on Why Everyone Should Consider Treating Their Herpes Holistically.

There are only three ways of managing herpes. You can manage your herpes through drug therapy or holistic therapy anchored with herbal medicine or you can decide to not treat your herpes at all. Drug Therapy has side effects that can be detrimental to your health, and does nothing to build up your immune system or improve your overall health. If you are sexually active not treating your herpes is unethical since you will be endangering others by not treating a life-long contagious viral infection not to mention that it increases your chances of becoming infected with human immunodeficiency virus (HIV), human papilloma virus, also known as genital warts (HPV) and other sexually transmitted infections. Holistic therapy has no disadvantages so it would seem to me to be the obvious choice.

1. Holistic Therapy can be just as effective, if not more effective, as drug therapy.

2. Holistic Therapy builds your immune system and helps you protect yourself against other sexually transmitted infections and immune related illnesses such as cancer - which drug therapy does not do.

3. Holistic Therapy helps you better cope with the emotional and psychological impact of having herpes which drug therapy doesn't even pretend to do.

4. Holistic Therapy is steeped in the ancient traditions of holistic and traditional healing from all world cultures - so it's getting back to your roots and re-connecting with nature in a satisfying and uplifting way.

5. Holistic Therapy helps you to grow and become a better human being and a better member of your community - who would ever claim that drug therapy ever accomplishes that!

Holistic Therapy for herpes is based on four simple ways

of supporting your immune system and yourself as a whole person. The first way is through eating an appropriate diet for herpes. The second is making some changes to your exercise routines and adding some creative visualization to give yourself mental and emotional support. Thirdly there are a few simple supplements that help your immune system with herpes, they are inexpensive and easy to find, they are; garlic, zinc picolinate, selenium (preferably from brewer's yeast), hemp seeds (not hemp protein) and lauricidin- only if you have frequent outbreaks, and only buy from http://www. lauricidin.com (I have no financial connection to Dr. Kabara so my advice is unbiased).

Lastly Holistic therapy requires real herbal medicine. You can make remedies yourself at home very inexpensively which I encourage people to try. You can get the remedies from me that I make from scratch like my grandmother did and my family has for generations, or you can get your medicine from your local qualified herbalist. Please do not buy quick fix gimmick solutions, you cannot manage herpes with l-lysine, you cannot manage herpes with D.M.S.O and hydrogen peroxide (in fact it's dangerous and illegal to do so) or other hoaxes like MMS or BHT. You cannot manage herpes with topical creams, gels, or essential oils.

This is a pitch for those who haven't given holistic healing a chance, to explore holistic healing and especially the message of making peace with the virus. Do not treat it like some cockroach you want to exterminate. Again I encourage people to make their own remedies or get on my protocol.

Because I don't believe in impersonal medicine, everyone who reads this book can request a consultation with me to find out more about my herpes treatment protocol. Ask questions and get some moral support from someone who's been there before and who cares, contact me at christopher. scipio@gmail.com.

Why Your Doctor May Be the Last Person You Want to Speak with About Herpes

Most doctors are uninterested and unsympathetic to persons with herpes. Doctors are busy seeing lots of patients and are making lots of money. Herpes is a disease very few doctors have taken an interest in as there is no glamour involved with herpes like with cancer or heart disease. There are no big charities or foundations with millions or billions for research, and it's incurable. Other than writing a prescription for an acyclovir-based drug there's not much else a doctor can do for persons with herpes. Very few doctors are going to invest the time and compassion in discussing the mental and emotional aspects of living with herpes. Very few doctors will want to discuss what's involved in safer sex.

Many doctors, and even a surprising number of dermatologists are not that competent at diagnosing herpes. Most doctors cannot accurately diagnose a herpes sore by visual inspection. I was misdiagnosed for two years by a series of doctors who not only visually inspected my sores but also took swabs and gave me false negatives. Herpes can appear in a wide variety of forms; the typical colony of pin-prick sized liquid-headed lesions, a single small pimple, a single-large pimple, a tear or slit in the skin like a fissure, various rashes, impersonations of ingrown hairs and skin-tags. If you suspect you have herpes insist on a type-specific blood test. The Western-Blot test is the most accurate one out, but there are others. Your local chapter of Planned Parenthood can help you get a test if your doctor is reluctant.

Many doctors are surprisingly uninformed about herpes. I spend a lot of my time correcting bad information given to my patients by their doctors. Some doctors are even still telling people that they cannot spread herpes to others when they are not having an outbreak. Many doctors also exaggerate the hype about asymptomatic shedding and overstate the effectiveness of drug therapy for herpes which aids the drug companies in their marketing efforts.

Most doctors give the public misinformation about the effectiveness of natural therapies for herpes. The medical profession, in alliance with the drug companies, has been discouraging the general public from seeking natural treatment for herpes by repeating the lie that there are no effective natural treatments for herpes. Drug companies don't want to spend the money to study natural therapies because they cannot patent such therapies. Governments won't spend the money because they don't want to validate safe, natural, inexpensive therapies which would compete with the expensive and highly-profitable drug therapies, despite the fact that the drug therapies cause negative side-effects. There have been dozens upon dozens of studies which demonstrate the merit of natural therapies for herpes including simple things like doing Hatha yoga regularly. Melissa Officinalis, Olive leaf, Garlic, Lomatium Dissectum, Prunella Vulgaris, Lauricidin and many other natural substances have been shown to be effective in clinical studies. I have seen over 170 citations of clinical studies about natural treatments for herpes. The scientific community and the medical establishment play games with the public by trying to invalidate these studies by saying that the sample size was too small for their liking or that they were conducted overseas and are somehow invalid.

Don't expect an unbiased opinion on natural medicine from your doctor. I have written before that asking a doctor to comment on natural medicine is like asking an atheist to comment on the bible, or asking a Muslim cleric to comment on the Talmud.

We don't need to rely solely on clinical studies to prove that natural medicine works. Natural practitioners have hundreds of years of clinical results with their patients to prove the effectiveness of their methods. If you treat patients and can see the results yourself over and over again, that is the most concrete way of evaluating natural medicine in my opinion. People can quibble over the results of studies but no one can tell my patients they haven't gotten better if they have.

Christopher Scipio
Homeopath/Herbalist
Holistic Viral Specialist
2015

Introduction:

My First Year with My Friend Herpes.
or
How I was Re-born a Modern-day Leper.

It was 1990, I was 25 years old and I didn't think my life could get any worse. I had just finished college and my financial situation was worse than dire. The country was in the midst of an economic depression. A long dismal winter had just given up the ghost and to top it all off I was in the middle of a horrific break-up with a vengeful girlfriend.

Of course it was pathetically naive of me to think that life couldn't get any worse and life wasted no time proving that fact. My relationship with this beautiful, vivacious, urbane woman had begun most promisingly. We had courted very romantically by letter and phone for six months before ever getting together. I was still at University when we first met and we were separated by a distance of about 1200 miles. We started off as friends and the love between us grew slowly with all the optimism and passion we expected. Sadly, what was so wonderful by distance was a nightmare up close. When my classes ended and I flew down to move in with her it took no time at all for things to go very, very wrong. Our sex life was hot despite the fact told me she had herpes. She told me that she could tell when she was getting an outbreak and as long as we refrained from having sex at those times, it was cool for us to have a natural unprotected sex life. I believed her, and she certainly sincerely believed this to be the case. She had only very recently gotten the disease herself from a man she had casually slept with who didn't tell her he was infected.

We got along in bed much better than we ever did out of bed; the tall beautiful fair-skinned princess and her tall, Black dread-locked artist. The sad fact was that we didn't get along at all. Instead of creating harmony, we created war. And I must say that I am to blame for much it. I was at a time in my life where my tolerance for certain things was very low and I was very angry about how the world was treating me and I certainly didn't enjoy the treatment I was receiving from my beloved - but I definitely contributed more than my fair share to the discord. Once we were in the same space together the chemistry between us was bad, bad, bad. The relationship ended after a mercifully short time leaving us scattered, raw and dumb-founded.

Two days after the notorious breakup we were reunited by a particularly cruel twist of fate. Less than 48 hours after swearing I would never see her again I was sitting beside her in the waiting room of a hospital. She was looking at me with a combination of guilt, sadness and white-hot enmity. I didn't know how to feel or what to say to her. I was floating around out in space trying to get a grip on the situation.

You see dear readers I was in the midst of what I would later find out to be my first herpes outbreak. It had started out as an itchy irritation on my foreskin but had quickly turned into a raging swelling colony of tiny lesions and I was overwhelmed by the pain and all the flu-like symptoms typical of first outbreaks. I had no idea what was happening to me. I do remember hoping at the time that it was anything but herpes or AIDS. I even considered syphilis or gonorrhea to be preferable. The doctors said they couldn't tell what it was that I had and insisted that my ex-girlfriend of two days come in with me so we could both be tested at the same time.

Even though we both hated each other at the time, I remember feeling sorry for her. I knew even then that if it proved true that she had given herpes to me, she would be devastated. So there we were with all those mixed emotions dreading the worse and hoping for the best.

The doctors tormented us by making us wait about a week before the test results would be back. They had taken a swab of my lesions and sent it off somewhere. When the phone call eventually came in the news was good. I had tested negative for herpes. The doctors said they still didn't know what it was that I had, that possibly it was just an infection of my foreskin from having rough sex. I was over the moon with relief and wasted no time in calling her to tell her the good news. For one brief moment we actually had something positive to share together. That test result was a big reprieve for both of us. Sadly and ironically it turned out only to be a reprieve for one of us.

To her credit she had been upfront with me. At the time I really had no idea what the implications and risks were. I was however prepared to take the risk; I just had no idea that this would literally be a very ironic last interaction in what had been probably the worst relationship both of us would ever have in our lives.

I went on with my life and forgot all about herpes. But herpes didn't forget about me, not for a second. I got another outbreak two months later and then another one a month later. The mysterious outbreaks settled down for a time but would always come back. I still couldn't get a diagnosis form the doctors. Two years later, I couldn't take it anymore and stormed into a different hospital demanding to know what was wrong with me. At this hospital the doctors were more competent and took one look at my penis and told me that it was obvious that I had herpes. They confirmed this with their own cotton swab test. There were no blood tests for herpes in Canada available at this point in history. They told me that false negatives were common for herpes because if there wasn't enough virus present on the skin at the time of the test, then you would get a negative result even though you had herpes. They told me there was nothing they could do for me and that I would have this disease for life and that my sex life would never be the same.

I wanted to call my ex-love and blast her for what had happened. I didn't have the heart to throw this in her face. So I never told her that she gave me herpes.

I do not possess the power to describe the world of pain and shame the eventual diagnosis of herpes would thrust me into. In many ways I felt like my life was truly over. I felt dirty in a way that I had never experienced before. Just saying the word herpes sent a chill through my whole body. The doctors were cold and unsympathetic. I couldn't discuss this with anyone in my conservative West-Indian family even though we were otherwise close. I didn't have anyone to talk to. Strange fatalistic fantasies went through my mind all day long, day after day. The mere thought of having to tell someone that I had this thing made me want to run for the cover of enforced celibacy.

I felt cursed like some Old Testament character. Sure I had been an asshole, not unlike most men my age, but I had definitely not been enough of an asshole to deserve to be punished by the Gods this way. This was definitely overkill in all meanings of the word.

My first realization after being able to admit to myself that I had herpes was that it was forever. No matter what I did or who I became I was never going to be a "whole" person. I was "marked" for life. I had joined an outcast caste. I was one of the many modern day lepers; those sad morally challenged people with herpes. I was a victim and I sure didn't like the feeling. What a burden to have to carry all the rest of my life.

Yes, I was now one of them. I had no real idea of what being one of them really meant. To find out would take years and many experiences both liberating and devastating.

Why am I telling you all of this? Part of it is narcissism to be sure. It's human nature to want your story preserved somewhere in the ether and this is my way of making sure that some people know what happened to me and how I felt about it. But the larger part of my motivation is for my own rehabilitation. I refuse to be a victim to this disease and to society's mean, irrational fear and loathing of those of us who are stricken with sexually transmitted diseases. I wasn't living a high-risk lifestyle - I got my herpes in the context of a monogamous relationship. But even if I had been doing high-risk activities, I in no way deserve to be scorned or ostracized because of it. The worst place to be when you have herpes is in the closet. If you want to feel like a leper and allow others to treat you like one, be my guest. I am determined not to live like that. Instead of being imprisoned by this disease, I decided to free myself. I am no longer afraid of saying the word and letting people know that I am one of "them". I have herpes but herpes doesn't have me. I am at peace with the virus and the virus is at peace with me. I am at peace with my place in this world and I have discovered the joy of encouraging others to liberate themselves from the stigma.

In part two of this Story, "Nine Years in the Wildness: My Personal and Professional Quest for a Holistic Herpes Treatment Plan", I chronicle how I transitioned from being a victim of herpes to being a Holistic Herpes Treatment Specialist and a herpes spokesperson. I was able to turn the biggest negative in my life to one of the biggest positives in my life and the journey is just beginning. We are truly living in a Herpes Nation with 60% or more of the general population in North America having either type one or type two herpes.

Chapter One:
Nine Years in The Wilderness:
My Personal and Professional Search for a
Holistic Herpes Treatment Protocol

It's a jungle out there.
I didn't realize how much of a jungle it was out there until I started to look for a natural way to treat my herpes.

For the first couple of years after being infected with herpes the only thing the doctors gave me was an acyclovir cream called Zovirax. It was expensive- about $50 for 5ml in 1993 dollars. I would put it on my penis anytime I felt the tingling that would signal an oncoming outbreak. It was supposed to stop the outbreak from coming, but it never did. It was also supposed to make my outbreaks less severe and heal faster. Perhaps it did for others but it never did for me. I got outbreaks three or four times a year and they would always be an eruption of a colony of pin-prick sized lesions in the same spot on my foreskin. It was painful and the lesions would be fluid-filled and would swell and… I'll spare you the rest of the gory details. Suffice it to say that it was two or three weeks of physical, emotional and spiritual hell for me. Being on my foreskin, my outbreak would always rub against the inside of my pants or my underwear- making things worse. Being from a born-again Christian background every time I got an outbreak I felt like I was being punished by God. Outbreaks always plunged me into a deep abyss of depression. During an outbreak it would be hard for me to think of anything else. I would be constantly pulling my pants down to check on the damage and I was desperate for anything that would help me stop this horror.

The desperation drove me to try anything that promised to help with herpes. Despite the fact that I was a struggling photographer barely able to support myself, I spent all my money on the Zovirax and all kinds of "treatments" for herpes.

I heard that olive leaf was good for herpes so I took olive leaf capsules and also broke open the capsules and applied the olive leaf to my skin before and during outbreaks. Unfortunately it didn't help much and sometimes seemed to make things worse.

I then heard about Camu-Camu (Royal Camu) an Amazonian berry touted as having thirty times as much vitamin C as an orange. They were advertising all over the place that this was a break-through treatment for herpes. It was expensive about $45 for 120 capsules, but I tried it and the only thing it broke through was my meager bank account.

I similarly tried everything else; lysine, D.M.S.O (which burned me), hydrogen peroxide, essential oils of melissa, hyssop and lavender, ice, cayenne pepper, red marine algae, cats claw, pau d'arco- you name it. The essential oils and the red marine algae helped for a short period of time and then lost their effectiveness altogether.

At the height of my desperation and despite my dislike of drugs, I tried Valtrex. The drug gave me intense migraine headaches from the first pill I put in my mouth. It also made my body feel weird in many other ways. So I was unable to even finish the $180 dollar bottle I bought.

I was completely lost in the wilderness. I had no one to talk to about my herpes. Everything I was reading on the internet and elsewhere seemed to completely contradict itself all the time. I often had this queasy feeling in my stomach like I was prey and these companies selling herpes treatments were like predators anxious to devour me.

I didn't know what to do and didn't know where to turn and this was me, from a family of ten generations of African-Caribbean herbalists! Herpes scared me right into the arms of the drug companies and they couldn't even help me.

I would like to say that I got a vision from my late grandmother, the well-respected herbalist and Shango Baptist priest, to point me in the right direction, but I can't say that because it didn't happen. What saved me from herpes hell was the AIDS crisis.

Being a fashion photographer I had many friends in the gay community and sadly some of them died from AIDS. AIDS by this time had taken much of the social pressure off of people with herpes because we no longer had the most horrible disease imaginable in the minds of the unsympathetic.

My friends in the gay community in Toronto started turning me on to some of the holistic protocols being put together to help give people with AIDS- an alternative to the wretched anti-viral drugs of the time like AZT. I started hearing about and sometimes meeting men who survived 7 to 10 years with full-blown AIDS without taking drug therapy. They told me they were controlling the virus through diet, meditation, vitamins, exercise and by changing their attitude. These men were a great inspiration for me. Some of them had been given only weeks to live by the doctors and here they were looking healthier than me.

I did at that time also turn to my memory of my grandmother's work with herbs and began planning on how I could develop a holistic protocol to heal my own herpes.

I threw away my Zovirax cream- which many doctors today admit is ineffective. I threw away my lysine.

I made two trips to China and spent six weeks there and started learning about Chinese herbs for skin problems.

It took me a year and a half but I was able to stop my own regular outbreaks by changing my diet, meditating (although I was never good at it), taking garlic and zinc picolinate and selenium and making some simple herbal formulas. These helped greatly but I think the most important thing I did was come out of the closet.

I started making peace with the herpes virus in me and started to confess my herpes status to my friends and lovers, something I had never been comfortable doing before.

This lifted such a heavy burden off of me. I felt, younger and lighter and whole for the first time since I got my first outbreak. I started to reject the notion that I was dirty or compromised by having herpes. I started to feel sexy and clean again. In short I liberated myself from the only experience of slavery I have ever known.

Treating Herpes Safely, Naturally, Effectively
Part One:
A New Holistic Approach to the Treatment of Herpes and Cold Sores

A million people or more will contract herpes 1 or 2 this year in North America alone. It's estimated that 60% of the population has herpes. A majority of the people with the disease are unaware that they carry the virus, making them much more likely to pass it on to others. With so many people affected by this epidemic, it's a wonder that herpes doesn't get more media attention. It's been labeled an incurable disease which left untreated can have serious consequences. Those consequences include the small risk of the death of an infant born to a mother having an outbreak during delivery and vast increase of one's chances of being infected with HIV or HPV.

The sad fact is that there's still a pervasive wall of shame and silence around this disease. People are much more likely to publicly declare their HIV positive status than admit to having herpes. There are numerous charities and foundations with their high-profile celebrity spokespersons leading the very public campaign of AIDS awareness and research. There's an ever-increasing amount of sympathy and support for AIDS victims from the general public. I challenge anyone to name a public spokesperson for herpes. Better yet, can anyone even name one single herpes charity? I'm sure they exist, but their public profiles are next to nonexistent. Have you ever seen a telethon to raise money for herpes research? It's inconceivable to me why herpes is treated as such a "dirty" disease. Is it the modern leprosy? I have worked with many herpes patients who do not tell their lovers of their status for fear of being rejected. I'm not sure what the answer would be to gaining more support and sympathy for the sufferers of herpes, but it's something we could all work on.

The Acyclovir family of drugs-including Valtrex and Famvir has been the long standing therapy prescribed by doctors for the treatment of herpes 1 and 2. Although the drug has proven itself to be somewhat effective in the reduction of the duration and severity of outbreaks when used episodically and in the suppression of some outbreaks when taken daily, this effectiveness can come with a steep price.

Acyclovir does not cure herpes, and must be taken indefinitely. Like many other drugs there are serious possible side-effects, including kidney dysfunction, toxicity in the nervous system, nausea, vomiting, diarrhea, seizures, confusion and tremors and severe headaches. Beyond these perhaps the biggest problem with taking these drugs for herpes is the false sense of security they can create, providing an excuse for some not to practice safer sex.

I have been using natural remedies to help people suffering with herpes for seventeen years now. One of the principle natural tools used in controlling herpes has been L-lysine-an amino acid that has been proven to reduce the frequency of outbreak in some people. Unfortunately L-lysine has now been shown to have its own serious side-effect. Since it's main action is to inhibit arginine in the cellular environment, the long term effect of taking L-lysine is the lowering of the body's immune function; which is a less than a desirable outcome.

A Comprehensive Program for Managing Herpes Safely and Effectively

Twenty-four years ago I contracted herpes myself in the context of a monogamous relationship. Being open-minded and desperate I tried drug therapy and immediately got migraine headaches for the first time in my life. It was clear that I had to find a natural way of managing the disease for myself since I was going to have it for the rest of my life and I needed a way of being able to resume my sex life without the dread of the likelihood of passing it on to others. In the next two years I tried every natural therapy available at the time. Frustrated from the lack of consistent and lasting results from most of the touted natural remedies for herpes, I started developing my own treatment program based on my family's multi-generational background as herbalists.

What I found through my experience is that herpes needs to be addressed on many levels. Nutrition and lifestyle changes and adjustments are necessary; equally, if not more important, are the deep shame and many psychological effects of the disease. Herpes also can change quite significantly during the course of someone's history so any protocol would have to be flexible enough to deal with the evolutionary nature of the presenting symptoms.

I also don't believe in the necessity of suppressive therapy for herpes. Unless you plan to be on Valtrex for life, suppression does nothing to strengthen your immune system nor does it stop the outbreaks from returning once you stop. My protocol is not designed to suppress outbreaks altogether but rather to lengthen the period of time between outbreaks and to shorten their duration and greatly lessen their severity. Some people have had their average duration of outbreaks reduced from 12 to 16 days to 1 to 2 days. Some people have been able to prevent most outbreaks from re-occurring

The protocol does not cure the disease and does not stop all symptoms from appearing. Even those who have been able to stop most of their outbreaks have experienced some mild infrequent outbreaks, many less than one per year, some far less than that.

After taking someone's case the protocol is adjusted depending on the strain of the virus, the frequency, location and duration of outbreaks, the relative health of the patient's self-esteem, and the relative level of stressors. Other things to consider are whether the client is male or female, length of time with the disease, etc. For most the protocol involves both internal and topical remedies. For all it involves combination therapy; I learned a great deal from studying how other natural practitioners were treating HIV, especially people who had both HIV and herpes or who had drug-resistant HIV. In North America many people with HIV also have herpes. Many of the same substances that are effective for HIV are also effective for herpes.

All of the substances in the protocol are from whole plants. Many of the plants are gathered by hand by herbalist friends and colleagues or are grown organically and lab-tested.

As of today I use over 170 different plants to treat herpes. Most are Chinese, Amazonian Herbs or Herbs from India- as these are the places where some of the most powerful anti-viral plants grow. The time of year and each patients specific symtpoms determine which of these plants will be combined in the forumlas I hand-make for them.

Living in Canada also allows me to have access to some of the greatest medicinal red marine algae and mushrooms in the world. I spent many years exploring which red marine algae and mushrooms are effective for my herpes patients and include them when needed in their protocol remedies. I love making remedies and I love connecting people to plants.

For those with regular symptoms there are self-hypnosis CDs that are part of The Protocol. Hypnosis has proven itself to be very effective in the treatment of herpes particularly when combined with other therapies.

Lastly, I counsel people to make peace with the disease; to not treat the virus as some ghastly invader, but to somehow dialogue with the virus and reach some kind of accommodation. The virus is an innately intelligent, motivated organism quite capable of surviving. The virus is just one of many, many micro organisms homesteading in our bodies. I encourage people whenever possible to make an agreement with the virus to allow the virus to stay, if the virus agrees to cause as little disruption to their life as possible. Above all else, do not be ashamed of having herpes. Have the courage to reclaim your self-esteem and never let yourself feel unworthy.

Why I am not Ashamed of Having Herpes

Why should I be?

I will not allow myself to be ridiculed, stigmatized or disrespected by others for having a disease. Disease is a natural part of life whether you are human, animal or plant. Nobody is exempt from disease, almost no one will live their full life without getting at least one sexually transmitted disease. These are facts.

Some people are afraid of diseases and those who have them. This is an ancient, primal fear, and one I understand well, but it doesn't excuse anyone from mean-spirited, ignorant behaviour towards those with diseases.

When I was a kid we made fun of "retarded" and "handicapped" people. I am deeply ashamed of that now, but children can be quite brutal. Adults need to hold themselves to a much higher standard.

Those who make sick jokes about herpes are not only aping the same mentality as those who make racist or sexist jokes, but they are also exposing their own lack of courage. It's much easier to ridicule the things you are afraid of rather than having the courage to face those fears. They are creating a stigma that causes millions of people with herpes unnecessary grief.

At least 60% of the population has herpes above or below the waist. 70% of the population will get HPV as genital warts or cervical dysplasia. 80% will get chlamydia at least once- most women will get it more than once.

All animals with backbones get herpes- including cats, horses, elephants and salmon. Most animals without a backbone get herpes- including worms.

Having herpes doesn't make me less moral, less attractive, less ethical, less worthy of respect, less sexy or less of a great catch, so why would I be ashamed to have herpes?

I am not afraid of my body. I know that sometimes I will get sick. I know that my faculties will decline as I age and that I am destined to die. This is the beauty of life- the contrast and balance between health and disease, between happiness and sorrow, summer and winter, fullness and emptiness, life and death.

I am a natural person; I am not ashamed or at war with any part of my body, including the herpes virus. I am at peace with the virus, my body and my place in this world as a person with a lifelong herpes infection.

I am most definitely not ashamed.

Nobody Else in the World has Herpes the Same Way You Do

I have said it millions of times. I have written it dozens of times, but I think it bears repeating because maybe the message isn't getting out as well as it needs to, so here we go: Nobody else in the whole wide world has herpes the same way you do.

Frequently people write to me confused and frustrated because their herpes symptoms are not following the stereotype of how herpes is supposed to be. People have heard that you are supposed to have fewer outbreaks the longer you have herpes. This is simply misleading and inaccurate. There are many factors that can make your herpes symptoms worsen at any point and time: you could have unprotected sex with someone else with herpes; you could get a secondary infection like HPV or bacterial vaginitis; you could impair your immune system with substance abuse; if you are a woman over 35 your hormone imbalance could worsen herpes symptoms, etc.

Herpes is an individual experience. It's almost useless to compare your symptoms with those of anyone else. Sure you could hunt down herpes photos online, but herpes sores can take on a variety of forms. They can look like a cluster of pin-prick sized lesions, or they can look like solitary pimples. They can look like fissures, or they can look like patches of rough skin or like ingrown hairs. Many MD's cannot diagnose herpes accurately by visual inspection and must rely on blood tests or swabs, and you would need to, as well.

Your diet, race, sex, age, lifestyle, emotional health, spiritual practices, sexual habits, exercise routine, genes, the virulence of the strain or strains you are infected with, and the environment around you will all affect your herpes symptoms.

So instead of comparing yourself to others with herpes, your time and energy would be better spent getting to know your own herpes better. Pay attention to your body and understand what triggers your symptoms. Make peace with your virus and do the inner work necessary to keep the virus dormant. Practice safer sex with a condom and my red marine algae antiviral sex gel. Strengthen your immune system and live a holistically healthy lifestyle.

Nine Stages of Dealing With a Herpes Diagnosis

Since no two people are going to get herpes the same way, and everyone's experience with the disease will be their own unique one, this will affect you on a mental and emotional level just as uniquely. I've noticed in my experience of treating herpes nine different stages that I've gone through myself and have seen others go through.

Shock:

Being told that you have herpes can be downright shocking. For myself I was told I had herpes when I was 25 years old. I was at the peak of my youth and health. I had just finished college. I definitely had a belief in my invulnerability. I felt almost immortal. I had never been sick before. Then I got slammed hard with the diagnosis. For months I was in shock. I couldn't process it. I had never spoken to someone before who admitted they had herpes. I couldn't believe that something like this could have happened to me. I believed in safer sex and had worn condoms all the time. I thought that herpes was something that only happened to dirty people, promiscuous people. I had gotten my fair share but was by no means promiscuous. I got herpes in a monogamous relationship where we had both been faithful to each other. Not only was I in shock for a great length of time, I was also numb and disorientated. This diagnosis had shaken me to the core and my world would never be the same again.

I eventually got over the shock of having herpes by facing the reality of it and learning everything I could about it and making it real and tangible for myself.

Anger:

This is the most common stage of dealing with herpes. I'm not surprised that many of the men who come to me are angry, but I'm shocked by how many of the women are and by how angry they are. Many women have a burning, white-hot anger over their herpes diagnosis. Many were betrayed by their lover/boyfriend/husband. Too many men don't tell their women that they have herpes or downright lie and say they don't. Too many men will say and do anything just to get laid or to get away with cheating on their woman. So women are especially angry if deceit or betrayal is part of their experience of getting herpes and it often is.

But even if a person wasn't lied to or betrayed, anger is still a stage experienced by almost everyone who gets herpes. Many people get angry at the virus itself thinking of it like some cockroach they want to crush. They hate the virus and want it dead and gone.

I was never angry at the virus per se, I was angry at my body for not protecting me from the virus and I was more angry about what having herpes was going to mean for the rest of my life. I was angry that I was no longer "clean." I used to take pride in being able to tell lovers that I was clean and had never had a sexually transmitted disease or a disease of any kind except for chicken pox. I was one of those rare kids that had never had a cold sore, neither had anyone in my family. I was a health freak, mostly a vegetarian who cooked my own food and took great care of my body. Now I was angry at having to tell people I was a leper and never again being able to enjoy the fruits of a disease free sexuality. I was angry every time I got an outbreak. It was a painful and embarrassing situation for me each and every time. My body

33

that I had taken such good care of was out of control and nothing I did could get it back under control.

I was very angry at the doctors who treated me. Those incompetents misdiagnosed me for two years telling me I didn't have herpes. Those were two years where I could have infected other people. The doctors, once they figured out that I had herpes, treated me like I was dirty and didn't want to spend even a minute talking to me about how to have safer sex with herpes, what to eat and not eat or what options I had for managing it.

Lastly I was mad at society for not doing anything to help educate me about the risks of getting herpes and how to protect myself. Herpes was never discussed during sex education classes in school, not even at college or university. I had never heard anything about it in newspaper or on the radio or television, there was no internet in those days but when I went to the library to look it up after finding out I had it- there wasn't any good information available there either.

I was one angry person for quite a long time and to make matters worse I didn't have anyone to talk to about it. All that anger just seethed inside of me, which of course triggered outbreak after outbreak. I didn't stop having outbreaks until I stopped being angry about herpes years later.

Bitterness:

Despite the fact that she had warned me that she had had herpes, I eventually became bitter towards the ex-girlfriend who gave me herpes. She had thought that she could predict when she was having outbreaks so she convinced me to have sex with her without condoms. She was working with what the doctors had told her, so she didn't deceive me at all. She just wanted to have her sex life back to the way it was before herpes. Still, I became bitter towards her for giving me the disease. I felt like she was a vampire that had turned me into a vampire without my permission and now there was no going back.

I eventually realized that staying bitter at the person who gave you herpes is an exercise in powerlessness. It keeps you in perpetual victim mode and keeps you tied to the past and to that person. To heal my herpes I wanted to be free of my past and free of my negative feelings towards that woman, so I let it all go. I had many dreams in which I had conversations with her. In those dreams I would put my arms around her or kiss her or just sit and laugh with her and we would make peace. We never made peace in real life, but letting go of her and my bitterness in my mind was enough to get me out of the bitterness ghetto, and I am no longer bitter at all towards her or about having herpes.

There is no future in being a victim so I encourage everyone to reject their bitterness when they are ready to.

Shame:

For many years just hearing or saying the word herpes was enough to make me cringe in shame. Every time I had to warn someone about my herpes it turned into a soap-opera melodrama with me crying or almost crying with shame.

I was so ashamed of having herpes. It sounded like the dirtiest word in the world, maybe even worse than the word nigger. It felt like the mark of Cain, like leprosy. I felt that there were all these clean disease-free people out there and that I was in this tiny persecuted minority of herpes people.

I was too ashamed to tell my friends or family, so I was left alone with my shame. Every time I would have an outbreak the shame would be multiplied dozens of times until that outbreak was finally over. Often I would stay home when I had an outbreak feeling unfit to even be in society.

Even after I had herpes for several years I would still hear people make nasty jokes about herpes and I would feel too ashamed to go after them for their intolerance. Sometimes I would look at personal ads and so many seemed to demand "disease-free" respondents only.

I got over my shame when I got tired of being a second-class citizen. I didn't want to feel ashamed of myself and I didn't want to be the subject of public or private ridicule. I decided to turn the biggest negative in my life into one of the biggest positives. I decided to go on the radio and to the print media and talk about my herpes and about herpes in general. I told people about the herpes treatment clinic I had established to help others like myself. The more I said the word herpes the easier it became to say. The more okay I was about my own herpes, the more okay others became about my herpes. It was an important lesson for me to learn in life. The outer world reacts to how you feel inside and you can't fake the funk. If you are not at peace with herpes and yourself, you will not have a happy experience with the disease. It's as simple as that.

Denial:

Denial is a stage easy to get lost in especially if you are not having frequent outbreaks. Denial is the most dangerous aspect of herpes as far as the community's health is concerned. People in denial about their herpes, especially men, are less likely to treat their herpes or warn others about their herpes or practice safer sex with an anti-viral gel and condom to help protect others from their herpes.

Nobody wants to have herpes. For the two years that the doctors misdiagnosed me I was praying that it was anything else than herpes. I would have gladly taken any other STD, except for HIV, instead of herpes.
It's easy to pretend that herpes is a pimple or an ingrown hair, or a mysterious rash or anything else.

Most people with so-called cold sores are pretending that they don't have herpes therefore they have become the main spreaders of the disease. Most of the 60% of the population that has herpes either got it from adults kissing them when they were kids or from people with cold sores (type 1 herpes of the mouth and face) performing oral sex on them.

Even scientists and doctors don't include people with herpes of the mouth and face when they report herpes statistics because they too are in denial that herpes is herpes whether you get it on the face or genitals. Whenever you see someone reporting herpes numbers and not including the 50-80% of the population that gets their herpes on their mouth and face, please ask them to stop being in denial and to stop lying to the general public about the scope of the worldwide herpes pandemic. The truth is that 60% of the population has herpes and that it's one of the biggest pandemics in world history. It is only possible to have a contagious disease that affects this many people not get discussed in the media because too many people are in denial.

Hope:

Once I stopped having regular outbreaks I became hopeful that I could live a herpes-free life. I knew the virus was always going to be in my body, but I began to hope that I could have sex without the morbid fear of infecting the person I was making love to. I began to hope that I didn't have to live in fear of another outbreak lurking around the corner, ready to spring out every time I ate a cashew or had a piece of chocolate. I began to hope that I could have sex without a condom as long as I used my antiviral gel and was sure I had not pressured my partner into taking risks they were not comfortable with.

Without hope life isn't worth living in my opinion but too many people sell false hope to people with herpes. The drug companies sell false hope to the public by promising to suppress 80% of viral shedding and to end regular outbreaks. This rarely happens. In the hundreds of herpes patients I treat a year, most of who have been on the herpes drugs, what I find is that only 40% to 60% of them experience the results claims by the medical community and for most of them those results will not be sustained for a prolonged period of time, for many the drug's effectiveness eventually starts to wane.

Worse are the snake-oil salesmen on the net; those anonymous companies unwilling to name themselves or even show their photos, promoting such dubious treatments for herpes such as D.M.S.O, hydrogen peroxide, BHT, MMS, magical topical formulas and worse. Every month there is a new miracle treatment for those gulliable or lazy enough to buy it.

Resignation:

At a certain stage it sinks in that herpes is for life. There isn't going to be a cure for herpes in our lifetime. There may never be a cure for this 140 million year-old disease.
Some people get resigned to having herpes and become complacent. As it is incurable, and because most people only experience mild symptoms, too many people feel that it is not worth the effort and expense to treat herpes.
After a time they even start to let down their guard about having safer sex. If you are still having regular outbreaks it's an ethical responsibility to treat your herpes and to practice safer sex, even if you are in a relationship with someone who also has herpes.

It isn't progressive or empowering to stay resigned or complacent about having herpes. It isn't even the best thing to do health wise.

Herpes is a gateway disease. Having herpes greatly increases your vulnerability to HIV, HPV and other sexually transmitted infections. Without treating your herpes and practicing safer sex you are playing Russian roulette with your body.

Gratitude:

Believe it or not I have learned to be grateful for having herpes. Don't get me wrong if I could go back in time and not have it I would. But I do have it and I'm grateful for it.

Herpes has helped teach me how to have more integrity. Herpes has forced me to take even better care of my body, mind and emotions. Herpes has made me come out of the closet and take on prejudice and intolerance head-on. Herpes has offered me an opportunity to help lots of people and make a living from helping them. Herpes has helped me understand holistic healing in a very profound way. Herpes has helped me understand the relationship between human beings and the micro-organisms that dominate the planet. Herpes has given me something in common with people I wouldn't have had much in common with and thus I have made some really special herpes friends I may not have otherwise crossed paths with. Herpes has helped me come to peace within myself and with the world around me. Having herpes has transformed me from an angry young Black man into a passionate but peaceful holistic warrior.

Yes it's true, I am grateful to the herpes virus in my body.

Peace:

Sadly, many people don't reach this most important stage of the herpes experience, but if you haven't it's your own fault. All that is required for peace is that you lay down your weapons and stop fighting. If you want to spend your life fighting an enemy you cannot defeat go ahead, history is full of tales of those fruitless campaigns like Napoleon's in Russia.

Tina Turner sings a song that goes "I don't care who's wrong or right, I don't really want to fight no more, it's time for letting go…"

Some people are so attracted to negativity, get such a rush out of it that they will never let it go. Everyone has the right to live how they wish to live. I will just say from my own story that peace is worth it. I didn't want to live a life of suppressed anger and end up with cancer or some other disease from holding all that bitterness in.

I wanted to be a positive force in this world instead of a negative one. I wanted to define myself and my relationship with herpes in a positive light, instead of being defined by others as some sort of sexually diseased outcast.
I decided to feel clean and sexy and moral despite having herpes.

I decided to embrace peace and all the fruits that come with it.

I am never going back to the other side.

The Parable of a Herpes Infection

We live in a wilderness. We were born in the wilderness and we lived on our parents homesteads as children. As adults we all struck out on our own when the time came and established our own homesteads.

Some of us came from parents who only used sustainable natural methods of farming. Most of us came from parents who only used man-made chemical fertilizers, pesticides and insecticides and who didn't fully respect the land and the environment around it. Some of our parents are still healthy; many of our parents are already paying a heavy price for their choices.

Some of us have chosen the natural way of working our farms, most of us have not. Regardless of how we farmed our homesteads, a calamity has befallen all of us. We and sixty percent of all the farms in the wilderness have been infested with a plague in our soil. The plague doesn't kill our crops but damages them and is contagious and can spread to any farms that have contact with our farm. There are two methods of dealing with this plague. The natural, sustainable method is to build back up your soil by rotating your crops, resting your soil, only planting organic heritage seeds, fertilizing your crops with seaweeds and other natural fertilizers, and using other natural methods of dealing with the plague such as planting protection crops. The natural method takes some hard work and time, but has us in complete harmony not only with our farm, but with nature itself. We are not stripping our soil of its nutrients so there is no need to use pumped up chemical fertilizers. In the natural method we understand that the plague is just part of the natural order of things, we are not mad at it, nor do we spend our time in the fields crying "why me?" or trying to kill the plague with dubious desperate schemes gleaned from the internet.

There is another way of dealing with the plague. A huge petrochemical company has developed a super expensive laboratory-made super-pesticide. This pesticide doesn't cure the plague but artificially keeps it in a state of suspended animation. The plague will still periodically devastate your crops, but the super-expensive pesticide has clinical studies to show that you will have fewer visits of the plague and will be less likely to pass the plague on to your neighbouring farms if you use this super-expensive highly-profitable artificial pesticide forever. The trick is, if and when you stop using the super-expensive pesticide the plague will return just as bad as before if not worse, and in the meantime- while using the pesticide, you've done nothing to build up your soil or learned how to farm sustainably, so you'll likely be worse off than before using the super-expensive pesticide.

Your common sense and intuition both tell you that there will be side-effects to using the super-expensive pesticide. Surely having this chemical on your food and in your air and water will have negative consequences, but the huge super-profitable petrochemical company assures you that you can trust them; they would never give anything to the general public that was unsafe, and that the side-effects are nothing to worry about. You also think in the back of your mind that you remember learning that previous laboratory made pesticides have all worked for a time but then usually eventually create pesticide-resistant strains of the plagues. The petrochemical company tells you not to worry about this either because so far there is no "evidence" that this super-pesticide will do that.

Out of either laziness, the compulsion to have an instant solution that requires little work on your part, or due to a lack of respect and faith in natural, sustainable methods, most of you decide to choose the super-pesticide, but then again you were under so much pressure to do so. The petrochemical company has lots of money to put advertising everywhere. The petrochemical company has all the local feed and fertilizer stores pressuring people into choosing the pesticide because they don't believe and respect the natural methods anymore. The petrochemical company also openly and also secretly sponsors and bribes almost all of the websites that give people information on how to deal with the plague. Many sites that look like they are independent are basically just fronts for the petrochemical company. The petrochemical company has many lobbyists and contributes lots of money to politicians so it influences the government to make it hard on anyone who promotes the natural/sustainable way of farming and managing the plague, although both the government and the petrochemical company know that the use of pesticides and insecticides and genetically modified seeds has a negative impact on the health of anyone eating the crops, and on the environment. The government still chooses to subsidize farms that use the petrochemical method.

You can manage your plague with chemical-therapy. It's expensive but faster and easier than sustainability. But there is always a cost to abandoning the natural way. Always.

I don't put my trust in big multi-national companies, nor in super-molecules created in labs by "smart" men in white lab coats. I prefer organic produce to factory farmed produce. I prefer organic free-range ethically farmed meat and chicken to factory farmed holocaust meat and chicken. I prefer fish ethically fished from nature than farmed fish. I prefer whole foods to factory processed foods. I prefer to cook than to eat out of a box. I prefer a woman who doesn't have silicone breast implants and botox injections.

I prefer living in harmony with nature and with myself. I am willing to do the work and put in the time, because ultimately, I am well worth it.

Chapter Two:

The Incredible, Mystical, Formidable Herpes Virus

You are one of the oldest forms of life on this planet. Yet you are not truly alive. Instead you walk the shadow-world between life and non-life.

You are feared by all, revered by none.

You infect all vertebrates and many invertebrates.
You are one of the driving forces in evolution. Your genes
have been incorporated into our genes.

You are a wonder of engineering and adaptability.

You are ruthless in your primal drive to survive.

You are the life-long uninvited guest in my body.

You are a red-hot wonder when active. Yet will lie dormant
for decades like a seed in the dessert waiting for an opportune
moment.

You are the Herpes Simplex Virus.

Memo To The Herpes Virus:
You need to hire a PR firm.

Although one of the least damaging viruses, milder even
than its relatives the chicken-pox/shingles virus and the
mono/glandular fever virus; herpes is feared, scorned, reviled
like almost no other disease in modern times. It's
a simple sexually-transmitted skin infection classified
as a minor disease in dermatological textbooks. But it's
sexually transmitted, and of course anything related to sex
in this sexually conflicted society comes under attack from
religious conservatives and those with unresolved sexual
hang-ups.

Herpes isn't one of the bad viruses that will kill its host. It
is a virus that merely wishes to take up permanent residence
in a host and remain dormant for long periods of time. Some
studies suggest that up to 70% of those infected by herpes

simplex do not have outbreaks that they can detect.

Herpes is a wonder of engineering. The debate in the scientific community about whether or not viruses are actually alive continues. Viruses lack the ability to survive and reproduce on their own. They are entirely dependant on having a host. The herpes virus is actually very similar to a computer virus in the way it behaves. Like a computer virus, herpes simplex penetrates into your hardware/body, re-programs your operating system/DNA to change the way your computer/body behaves and make billions of copies of itself. Viruses come close to fitting the definition of being alive but they stay on the boundary between life and ab-life. Viruses can grow in dead human cells and even have the ability to bring them back to life. Viruses can even stage their own resurrection. Even if you manage to destroy massive amount of a virus in your body, if there was more than one copy of the virus in any one cell, the virus can resurrect itself by playing Dr. Frankenstein, piecing together parts from more than one dead virus to create a new living whole virus.

The herpes virus, like no other virus I know of, has the ability to compel the host cell it has invaded to change it's shape and turn itself into a tunnel to the next healthy cell, so that herpes can move from cell to cell without exposing itself to your blood stream. This way your immune system has no chance of detecting and destroying it.

Just as impressive is the strategy the virus employs of only sending 50% of active virus during an outbreak to the surface of the skin. The other 50% of the activated virus it sends to infect uninfected cells. Thus it is never in danger of being wiped out of your body.

Viruses have been one of the key players in the evolution of humans and other animal life. When a virus has infected us in the past, if it has any genes which are useful to our evolution, those genes have been incorporated into our genome. When that same virus mutates, again, if there are any useful new genes, our bodies have (in our evolutionary past) incorporated those new genes into our DNA. Since viruses mutate faster than we can, they have had a profound influence on how we have evolved, as have bacteria. Viruses have had more of an effect on our evolution than climate change or other changes in our environment since those changes will always happen much more slowly than the mutation of viruses and bacteria. Some scientists believe that viruses created multicellular life on this planet to have hosts.

The word herpes comes from the Greek "to creep". Herpes was certainly an issue even to the ancient Greeks. Herpes can indeed creep from cell to cell undetected by the immune system. Herpes can creep from one outbreak location to others. Herpes does indeed creep from an infected person to an uninfected person. Herpes has been around for at least 140 million years and will be around long after we're gone from this planet. We still don't know a great deal about the herpes simplex virus. I have no doubt that as we get to know this virus better and better, it will become harder not to acknowledge it as an engineering marvel, a great survivor and evolutionary instigator.

Chapter Three:

Why Everyone Who Thinks They Don't Have Herpes Needs to Get a Blood Test

I have herpes, don't you?

You don't?

Are you sure?

I wouldn't be so sure if I were you.
Unless you have had a recent type-specific blood test to test for the presence of herpes simplex antibodies you cannot say with any certainty that you don't have herpes.

You think that only 20% of the population has herpes?

Think again.

You may have heard that one out of every five people has herpes, but that number is untrue and a distortion of the facts. The truth is that at least 60% of the adult population has herpes simplex.

You see some people, for reasons known only to them, decided to exclude people who get herpes above the waist, people who get so-called "cold sores" on their mouths and faces, from the herpes statistics commonly reported in the media, reporting only the percentage of people who get herpes below the waist, so-called genital herpes. This makes no sense at all since the scientific literature doesn't classify herpes simplex 1 (cold sores) as a different disease as herpes simplex 2 (genital herpes); but rather as two different types of the same disease, and since many of the new cases of herpes of the genital area are actually caused by people getting herpes simplex 1 on their genitals from oral sex. There really is no such thing as "cold sores". It is herpes simplex 1 of the mouth or face. And those who have it need not be in denial- pretending that it's anything other than herpes simplex. The truth is that you can get herpes simplex 1 on almost any part of your body including your nose, your elbows, your fingers, your stomach, your genitals, your anus, etc. The truth is that herpes simplex is herpes simplex and it is misleading to not include the people with herpes simplex 1 in herpes statistics.

Somewhere between 20 and 25% of the population get their herpes sores below the waist and somewhere between 50 and 80% of the population gets their herpes sores above the waist. If you factor in the number of people who have both herpes 1 and 2 at the same time, you are left understanding that at least 60% of the population has herpes simplex. Which rings true when you consider that 70% of the adult population has had HPV (genital warts or cervical dysplasia) and that 80% of the adult population has had Chlamydia at least once.

This is the reality of our times. There is almost no adult who has had more than six sex partners who hasn't caught a sexually transmitted infection. Including yourself. Including myself.

What? You say you've been tested before for sexually transmitted diseases and are clean?

I wouldn't be so sure. Herpes and HPV are almost never included in routine testing for sexually transmitted infections. Some doctors have the attitude that "Almost everyone tests positive for herpes so why bother testing". Unless you have specifically asked for a type-specific blood test for herpes, such as the Western Blot test, you have probably never had an accurate herpes test. Swabbing for the presence of herpes can and often does render false negative tests- I know that from personal experience. The doctors told me twice that I didn't have herpes before accurately testing me positive for herpes- although I had already had a very obvious primary outbreak.

I strongly encourage you to get a type-specific blood test for herpes if you believe that you don't have herpes, or are unsure of your herpes status. If you test negative for herpes, it will allow you to make some decisions regarding safer sexuality, to help keep you herpes free for the rest of your sexual history. If you test positive for herpes it will allow you to decide to treat your herpes and make safer sex choices to help you to not infect others and make this epidemic worse. Not only is it the ethical thing to do it is also the sane thing to do since herpes makes you more vulnerable to HIV and HPV. If you don't know, you won't get treatment. Knowledge is empowering. Denial is irresponsible.

What? You say you are sure you don't have herpes because you haven't had an outbreak?

Wake-up! Most people with herpes, maybe up to 70% don't get noticeable outbreaks. You may be having sub-clinical (subtle) outbreaks or may be shedding virus asymptomatically (without symptoms). You could be infecting others with herpes without knowing it.

Don't be afraid of getting a herpes test. Herpes can be effectively treated by a combination of diet, stress reduction and herbal medicine or by drug therapy. There is no cure but it is possible to go years between outbreaks.

I still believe that most people when given a choice prefer to do the right thing. Getting tested for herpes is the right thing.

Chapter Four:

The Demonization of Genital Herpes

Those of us who have so-called "genital herpes" are caught between a rock and a hard place. On one hand we are ostracized by the minority of the population (about 40%) who don't currently have herpes simplex in their body, which is bad enough, but more cruelly we are often isolated by our fellow members of the herpes community who have so-called cold sores (herpes simplex 1 of the mouth and face). Frankly the lack of support from the majority of the population who have cold sores bothers me far more than the stigma placed on me by unsympathetic members of the uninfected population. After all they don't know what it feels like to have herpes, so I can cut them some slack. But for those of you who have cold sores and continue pretending that you don't have herpes and who distance yourselves from those who have their outbreaks genitally rather than facially: shame on you. If it wasn't for your unwillingness to come to terms with the reality of your herpes infection, the herpes community would be a more united majority of the population far more empowered to boldly go out into the community and reject the unjust and irrational stigma placed on people with herpes.

Sixty percent of the population has herpes. We are living in a herpes nation. There is no reason for us to be a despised minority. If we were more united and more out of the closet we would be in a much better position to inspire understanding and support from those who do not have herpes. We would be better able to educate young people on herpes prevention and herpes awareness. We would be better able to reach out to the people with herpes who have had their self-esteem devastated.

So-called cold sores are herpes. I have had too many people in my clinic and through the internet say to me, "I don't have herpes, I've never had a STD, but I do get these cold sores on my lips."

Herpes is herpes whether you get your outbreaks above the waist or below the waist. It's true that people with type 1 herpes of the mouth and face often have fewer outbreaks than people with herpes type 2 of the genitals, but it is also true that herpes of the mouth and face is just as contagious if not more so than genital herpes. It is also true that many people with type 1 herpes of the mouth and face shed virus without symptoms and are giving many people type 1 herpes on their genitals from oral sex. It is also true that herpes of the mouth and face can spread to parts of the body that genital herpes rarely ever spreads to including the nostrils and into the brain, the hands and fingers, down the esophagus and into the stomach, into the eyes, and elsewhere.

For those who don't have herpes and give people with herpes a rough time, I really have no words for you. If you believe that having genital herpes is an indication of promiscuity or moral deficiency, then you are probably too far-gone for anything I say here to reach you. And for the record I don't think there's anything inherently wrong with promiscuity. I got my herpes in the context of a monogamous relationship, but I wouldn't feel bad about myself if I had been infected by herpes through promiscuity. How you got herpes is irrelevant. Herpes is a virus. Viruses have different strategies for gaining access to our bodies. A virus that chooses sex as it's preferred method of infection is less scary to me than an airborne virus that indiscriminately devastates huge populations in a matter of days.

Jesus said "let he who is without sin cast the first stone." I say let he or she who is without a virus cast the first stone. Between the Chicken-Pox virus (a member of the herpes family), the Epstein-Barr virus (another member of the herpes family), the HPV virus (genital warts and cervical dysplasia) and Herpes Simplex there is virtually no adult reading this article who doesn't currently have a virus in their body and except for the HPV virus, these viruses are lifelong infections and that's without even discussing bacteria, fungi, yeast, and protozoa.

Herpes has been around since the time of the dinosaurs and affects almost every single mammal including cats and elephants. In fact cats and elephants are dying of herpes. I know that cats can be randy but I have never heard of anyone accusing elephants of being promiscuous. If anyone has ever seen an elephant orgy let me know so that I can print a retraction.

When someone has the integrity and courage to tell you that they have herpes they are making themselves vulnerable to you. How you react can often either crush them or help set them free from a prison of shame. I believe that most people are intelligent and compassionate. Please treat people with herpes with the compassion and understanding we deserve. We are the same people we were before we got herpes. We are no less moral, no less attractive, just as good in bed, just as good of a friend or son or daughter or brother or sister as we were before we got herpes. When someone tells you they have herpes, if you treat them unsympathetically it only discourages them from telling others about their herpes in the future, which isn't a good situation for anyone. When someone tells you they have herpes it's an opportunity and challenge to you to show that you are not prejudiced and mean-spirited. It is a chance for us all to create more love and understanding.

For those of us who have genital herpes - don't buy into the lies and myths that make you ashamed and marginalized. You can choose not to let herpes define you and dominate your life. No one can take away your power and dignity except for yourself.

When someone gives you a bad time for having herpes instead of dwelling too long in anger or sadness, just "forgive them for they know not what they do". Embrace all the beauty and love around you and if there isn't enough beauty and love, create it. You are a human being equipped with infinite potential for loving and appreciating the wonders of this world.

How Easy is it to get Herpes from Oral Sex?

Because of the popularity of oral sex many people who have genital herpes have type 1 not type 2. Type 2 herpes prefers to be in your genital area but can also be on your face, although this is rare, and yes you would likely in this situation only have a primary outbreak and may never again see symptoms.

Anumber of people have both type 1 and type 2 herpes at the same time.

The only way to tell if the herpes you have on your genitals is type 1 or type 2 is to have it diagnosed with a swab. You cannot assume that just because you have herpes on your genitals that it is type 2.

Some information claims that type 1 infections of the genitals don't produce many outbreaks. This is a myth. No two people get herpes the same way and there are many factors which will determine how many outbreaks you get and how severe they will be.

If you have type 2 herpes on the genitals and someone performs oral sex on you, there is a slim chance that they will get type 2 herpes orally. If you have type 1 herpes on your genitals there is a much better chance that someone can then get type 1 of the mouth from you assuming they don't already have a type 1 infection of the mouth.

If you have type 1 herpes of the face, and please don't be in denial by labeling it as "cold sores," be aware that there is a substantial risk of you infecting others when you perform oral sex on them, and that the risk exists whether you are having symptoms you can notice or not. Just because you are not having an "outbreak" doesn't mean you are not contagious. If you have ever had a cold sore in your life, it means you have a life-long herpes infection no matter how long it's been since you have had an outbreak. You should avoid intimate contact with anyone when having any itching, tingling, burning or numbness anywhere on your face.

There are no clear numbers on what the actual statistical

risk is. I encourage everyone to consider lowering the risk by avoiding intimate contact during any possible symptom of the virus being active (itching, tingling, burning, or numb sensations anywhere below the waist), treating their herpes daily with real herbal medicine from a herbalist or with drug therapy and practicing safer sex with a condom and an anti-viral gel, http://www.antiviralgel.com.

Also keep in mind that according to statistics it is three times easier for a man to give herpes to a woman than for a woman to give it to a man, and that herpes infections are higher in the African-American and Hispanic populations than it is in the Caucasian population. I am Black myself, so I always want to encourage my brothers and sisters of colour to help get the message out to our communities about herpes awareness and the need to practice safer sexuality.

Herpes and Natural Childbirth

There's a lot of misinformation being circulated about the risk of a mother infecting her infant during natural childbirth. Neonatal herpes infection is a serious and sometimes fatal problem, but it is also a rare one. There is less than a 1 in 5000 chance of it happening. Through the use of Natural Medicine, hypnotherapy and Valtrex during the last month of pregnancy almost any woman who wants a safe, natural childbirth can have one.

The medical system pressures women to have c-sections which are less healthy for their babies, so that the risk of malpractice suits are reduced, and so doctors don't have to miss their regularly scheduled golf games to deal with the unpredictability of when a baby is ready to come into this world.

There are also effective Natural methods to help a man greatly reduce the chances of infecting his uninfected female partner during her pregnancy or during their attempts at conceiving a child.

Chapter Five:

Healing Herpes with Self-Love

When I was a boy we lived in the Ghettoes of Toronto, Canada. We had just immigrated from Trinidad and Tobago. My mother struggled to raise four of us on a waitress' salary. There was chaos and self-destruction all around us. Many of my playmates are no longer among the living. None of this touched us; we were living a different life. My mother was a church-lady. She was strong and resilient and strict. All of us grew up in the church. The church kept us insulated from most of the horrors of poverty.

The church still has its influence on me. I feel it and walk it everyday and I am happy for it. I learned about love in the church. Not the love you see on TV and in the movies; a bigger love, a deeper love. That's the one sermon from our Jamaican female pastor that I remember the most. When I was 13 she spoke about love. Jesus was all about love, He was love, and He is love.

Bryan Ferry from Roxy music sings "Love is the drug that I

need to score". I disagree. I don't believe that love is a drug, an intoxicant. That sounds more like infatuation to me. I believe that love is a medicine. The Medicine. For those of us in the sixty percent or more of the population with the herpes simplex virus Love is the most powerful healing tool.

Sarah McLachlan who went to my alma mater, The Nova Scotia College of Art and Design, sings "Your love is better than ice cream, better than anything I've ever had". I would sing instead that "My love is better than Valtrex, better than Famvir or anything I've ever had". Don Miguel Ruiz writes that "healing requires the truth, forgiveness and self-love. With these three points the whole world will heal". I will write about all three in this brief piece.

Figures vary widely but it cannot be disputed that between 50% and 80% of the population has herpes simplex 1 and between 20% and 25% of the population has herpes simplex 2, so if you factor in the number of people who have both types, the minimum number of people who have herpes simplex has to be at least 60% and is likely more. This is important because the message needs to get out to people with herpes that they are not part of some marginalized minority. If you have herpes you are part of a herpes nation that is a majority of the population. It is common and normal to have herpes. It is becoming uncommon not to have herpes. It is long past time for people with herpes to come out of the closet and speak up about herpes to help educate the people who don't have herpes and to put a human face on this disease. The stigma only exists because of the shame people with herpes have agreed to carry. There is no need for this, no reason for this. Shame is not a product of love.

It makes no sense to me to be ashamed of getting a virus

from an act of lovemaking or kissing rather than getting a disease from self-abuse or catching an air-borne virus from riding on a subway train. Some people do not love sex and therefore wish to denigrate anything that has to do with sex especially sexually transmitted infections. I learned a long time ago in church that true love is accepting and forgiving and inclusive. People with herpes are not lepers and need not allow themselves to be treated like lepers.

The truth is also that there is no cure for herpes and one isn't likely in our lifetime. So herpes is a lifelong viral infection. The truth is that most people who have herpes don't know it because they have never had a type-specific blood test for herpes either out of fear or lack of awareness. (Herpes tests are not normally part of a STI screening panel, so unless you demand one you may never get one.) The truth is that people with herpes can be contagious even when there are no warning signs of the virus being active; so safer sex is something that ought to be considered. The truth is that a person with herpes who does not make peace with the emotional and mental consequences of having herpes will not be able to manage their herpes as effectively as someone who does regardless of how much Valtrex or Famvir they take.

Forgiveness. Some people with herpes are still angry and resentful with the person who infected them. I can understand this because I hear so many stories. So many people are infected by people who didn't warn them of their herpes status. Many people are infected by unfaithful partners. Some have been raped.

It's natural to be angry and bitter when given a life-sentence like herpes. It took me a long time to let go of my negative feelings about my own infection. Everyone is living their own distinct experience with herpes. And I say most sincerely that sooner or later, and I hope that it's sooner, there must come a time to forgive and let go if you want to be healthy with herpes. Hanging on to the negative feelings not only damages you physically and otherwise, often causing more outbreaks, but it binds you to the past, which you will never free yourself from until you forgive.

Forgive the person who gave you herpes if you can. And if you cannot, keep trying until you can. But more importantly, forgive yourself. I treat so many people in my holistic herpes clinic who are continually punishing themselves for having herpes. They are angry at themselves thinking that they could have been smarter. They are full of regret and self- recriminations. This is not love. Love forgives, love understands.

Be good to yourself; be gentle and loving and patient as if you were your own child. Forgive yourself and reclaim your self-esteem and self-love.

Do you love yourself? Do you really? If you have herpes and love yourself how would you act? Would you be ashamed of your herpes? Would you stop dating and deny yourself love and sex just because you have herpes? Would you be sitting in a vortex of anger and resentment towards the virus? Or would your life be all about love and peace and balance?

If you loved yourself, how would you eat? Would you smoke cigarettes and take recreational drugs, would you drink coffee knowing that it's a trigger for your herpes and bad for your health all the way around?

If you loved yourself and loved others would you practice

safer sex with a condom and/or anti-viral gel to help protect your loved ones from your herpes? Would you practice safer sex to protect yourself from other sexually transmitted infections? Would you perhaps be motivated to speak out and try to educate others on how to deal with herpes if they have it or how to protect themselves from herpes if they don't, especially the young people who are just starting to explore their sexuality? If you loved yourself would you be afraid to warn your sex partners about your herpes status? The bible says that "true love casteth out all fear".

You were born with the right to be happy and to enjoy your life and your health to the fullest; having herpes changes none of this.

Chapter Six:

There Are No Quick-Fixes for Treating Herpes

Most of the true treasures of this world lay in the depths of things. If you were to content yourself with superficial things, think of what you'd be missing. If you only swam on the surface of the water you'd miss the wonders below. If you only ate the skin of fruits and vegetables you'd be in a sorry state. If all you ever read of a book were its first few pages, or if all you ever wanted to see in a film were the trailer, well you'd certainly be missing the big picture.

There are no quick fixes for herpes. The virus lives deep within you in the core of your nerve cells. It has access to all the thoughts and feelings that course through your body.

When you are in equilibrium, the virus is likely dormant; when you are out of balance, angry, scared, anxious, and ashamed the virus is likely going to be active.

To truly manage your herpes in a holistic way you have to take a deep personal inventory. What are your triggers? Are you at peace with the virus' permanent presence in your body? Have you been successful in rejecting the superficial and mean-spirited stigma placed on people with herpes and regaining all the self-esteem and confidence you lost when you found out you had herpes? Are you living a life of integrity by informing your potential romantic partners beforehand of your herpes status and doing your best to manage your herpes so that you are less likely to infect others? What are you willing to start doing to manage your herpes better? What are you willing to stop doing to manage your herpes better? Are you fixated on the negative aspects of having herpes or are you looking at the brighter side of things?

Once an unflinching personal inventory is taken it's possible to see the whole picture of having herpes. There are no completely negative or completely positive experiences in life. Herpes doesn't have to be a completely negative experience. There are positive aspects to having herpes.

Herpes can act like a barometer which sends you a warning when you have become too far out of balance.

Having herpes can be like a litmus test to show you who really cares about you. If after telling someone you have herpes they are less interested in pursuing a romantic and sexual relationship with you they didn't care enough about you to begin with. If after telling someone who is a friend or family member that you have herpes and you feel their lack of support, then you more clearly see where you stood with them all along.

Having herpes challenges your personal integrity. It challenges you to tell an uncomfortable truth to lovers for their own protection and challenges you to take measures to protect the health of others.

If you have never experienced what it is like to be scorned or be prejudiced against because of something out of your control, herpes helps you experience that reality so that you can sympathize better with other discriminated against people in our society.

Having herpes is a cold slap of humility in our all too arrogant existence as human beings on this planet. We have been taught by some of our religions and philosophies that we are the dominant force on the planet when in reality microbes have always been dominant and continue to be dominant. As I have said in other writings: we are a sideshow, most of the real action in this world happens on a microscopic level. We are a home to hundreds if not thousands of viruses, bacteria, fungi and protozoa. We could not digest food without the hundreds of bacteria in our mouths and intestines, we are colonized by microbes, most are beneficial or neutral, and some are harmful. Maybe with more humility we would be less likely to abuse the plants, animals and environment around us and see the bigger picture.

Staying in healthy balance with your own thoughts and emotions including making peace with the herpes virus is the most important step in managing herpes in a healthy holistic way. Herbal medicine, drug therapy, supplements, yoga, hypnosis, etc. can all help, but going deep within and creating peace and harmony in your life is the key.

Herpes: The Great Illuminator

Herpes can be a great illuminator.

When you are having an outbreak or herpes-related symptoms it can bring to the surface some of your deepest, darkest fears, insecurities and neuroses.

Some of the fears that my patients tell me that come up most often are insecurities about body image, memories of past sexual abuse, fear of not being desired or of being unattractive, fear of rejection, fear of infecting others, fear of ridicule and fear of being outed.

If you were struggling with your body image before having herpes, having outbreaks sends that fear right up into the stratosphere. This is the proverbial double-whammy. For some people until they make peace with their feelings about their body they will not have the virus under control. For others, until they make peace with herpes, having outbreaks will make the schism between themselves and their body much worse, and there will be no reconciliation between their bodies and themselves until they make peace with the virus first.

For those who were the victims of past sexual abuse or who were coerced into sex-work as young people, having symptoms of outbreaks can bring some ugly, terrifying or emotionally paralyzing feelings up to the surface, some of them long-buried. If the person was infected with herpes as part of the sexual abuse or exploitation, that adds another huge layer to the issue. This is the most daunting of the herpes illuminations, but it is better to have this illuminated and on the surface than repressed. Herpes can provide an opportunity to understand and work on this issue. Holistically healing your herpes can help change your relationship with yourself in an empowering way which can be part of a larger programme of healing these past wounds and vice-versa.

It is very challenging, obviously, to feel attractive and desired when having regular outbreaks or symptoms; this is one of the many reasons why having a supportive, understanding partner or partners is crucial for someone with herpes and why I encourage people to let go of anyone they are having an intimate relationship with who isn't completely supportive and understanding.

As human beings we tend to fear rejection more than any other fear. The advertising industry is largely propelled by reinforcing this fear in order to sell everything from antiperspirants to plastic surgery. It is especially crushing to be rejected for something you have no control over such as race, height or having herpes. Twinned with this fear of rejection is a fear of ridicule. There are a number of cruel people out there (thankfully only a small minority) who have said and continue to say harsh things about people with herpes. Most people are far more loving and tolerant than this but the fear of being ridiculed like the fear of rejection can get blown way out of proportion.

The fear of infecting others in and of itself can trigger symptoms and outbreaks. This is a healthy fear insofar as it can be a motivation for treating your herpes and practicing safer sex, but you should not allow it to become an overwhelming fear, or it may get in the way of reclaiming your sex life -which is a important step in living a holistically healthy life with herpes.

We could all make the fear of being outed a thing of the

past by coming out of the closet and talking about herpes, educating the general public about herpes and herpes prevention and by claiming our place in the sun as a majority of the population, but because we don't do this, we have imposed upon ourselves the status of a dis-empowered, ashamed community. I am always amazed by how far some people will go to not have to out themselves as a person with herpes. People have the right to keep their private lives private, but many of the people in the public arena who are willing to admit to me in private that they have herpes won't admit it in public, and this includes radio and television talk show hosts, porn stars, sex-educators, health-care workers, etc.

Until gays and lesbians started coming out of the closet in the 60's and 70's they had no rights or influence in this society, and so it will continue to be for us until we decide to change.

No matter how well you feel that you are doing on the emotional, mental and spiritual levels in dealing with herpes, it won't be until you are tested by outbreaks and symptoms that you will know where you truly are. Herpes is the great illuminator shining a piercing light on your deepest and darkest fears and insecurities related and un-related to "the gift."

Chapter Seven:

A Message For Women With Herpes
Herpes/Her-Peace

In my experience as a clinician it became apparent almost immediately that herpes is a very different disease for women than it is for men. It is easier for a woman to be infected with herpes than it is for a man. Women tend to experience more severe symptoms than men. Women are more likely to feel stigmatized by having herpes since we still live in a culture where many people (including many women) expect women to be purer than men. We embrace "bad boys," but we tend to punish "bad women". My three years of research with sex workers proved this point over and over again to me.

Women are more in touch with the forces of the universe than men are. Women tend to be the ones in any culture that maintain balance and hold families together. Women give birth to life and nurture life. Too many men destroy life: human life, animal life, plant life.

In many societies it has been the women that have preserved the healing knowledge of the local plants. This is true in my African-Caribbean culture.

If you are a woman who has herpes it's vitally important that you use your feminine instincts to make peace with the virus, reject any notion of yourself being dirty or compromised by having herpes, and reach out to your community for support and love. Some people ridicule the notion of making peace with herpes and write to me asking me how to make war on the virus. I always tell them that one of the fundamental rules of the art of war is to never fight a war that you cannot win.

Some people are inclined to be negative. They prefer to be angry and resentful and bitter towards the virus, towards the person who gave it to them, towards life, even towards me for even suggesting that making peace with herpes is possible. They prefer to say no when they can say yes. These people never do well with managing their herpes holistically. These people rarely experience the fullness of health and happiness.

Herpes lives in the base ganglion of your nervous system. If you have type 2 herpes it's right there in the sacral region of your spine. Herpes is tapped into every major nervous system in your body. Herpes can feel when you are unbalanced and negative and will respond by activating itself and it can sense when you are balanced and at peace and will tend to stay dormant.

I have only had one outbreak in the past four plus years because I am at peace with the virus in my body and with my body and with my life and with my community. I live a positive life. I enjoy this gift of being alive. I am happy. I don't need to take any supplements or remedies any longer to control my herpes. The peace and balance in my life has proven to be the most effective medicine ever.

Without peace and balance herpes will be the least of your problems. You will be more vulnerable to cancer and heart disease and everything else.

There's too much trouble in this world already. I encourage you to make your own life into an oasis of love and harmony. Sound too easy? You are a human being with virtually unlimited power and potential. You can make almost anything you want to happen - happen, if you believe and if you do the work.

Messages for My Black Brothers and Sisters with Herpes.

To All my Sistahs with Herpes.
I love you.
I straight up love you.

You are the noblest, proudest, most beautiful creatures ever born.
The true queens of this earth.
You carry us all with your every step.
You are the song of Solomon.
You are the taking in breathtaking.

Hold your heads high my Sistahs with Herpes.
Did you think this virus diminished you?
Did you think I would reject and leave you crying by the river?
Did you think that the sun and moon fell out of love with you?

You have faced and face far greater burdens than this one.
You have survived them all.
No overseer's whip, or racist slur or outbreak can rob you of what's truly yours.
The inheritance of Josephine and Billie and Sojourner.

Don't you hide away in some corner,
when the world needs your majestic light more than ever.
Don't suffer in silence,
when you possess the most powerful voice ever known.

It won't be Joshua's trumpet blowing down this wall of shame,
It will be the righteous chorus of my Sistahs ululating.

Rise up my Sistahs,
Sing and be free.

To All My Black Brothers

We are the true Kings of this earth. The fathers of mankind.
We were the first, the Adams. As we emerge from a 400 year
old nightmare, we must look into each others faces and see the
truth.

Let's stand tall like the warriors we were born to be. Let's
walk this earth like lions. Let's protect those who we love.
Let's stand up and be real. Let's banish this cloak of shame
and speak truthfully about our herpes infections.

When we lie or hide we let the nation down. When we
unreasonably refuse to wear condoms to protect our loved
ones, we weaken our nation.

We are twice as likely as whites to get herpes, not because
we are promiscuous for I don't buy into that lie, but because
we don't educate and empower ourselves to protect our own
precious bodies.

Our stress and poor nutrition add to the mix. As does an
appetite for self-destruction.

We were enslaved for our bodies and lynched because of our
bodies. We are worshipped in the sports arenas because of our
bodies, but we need to take back our bodies. We are no longer
beasts of burden. To re-claim our place in the sun we must
respect and revere our bodies. To be able to live our full life-
spans and produce healthy and happy future generations we

need to re-invest in our bodies, our minds and our souls. There is an ancient voice calling out for a new Black man to rise from the ashes, better and greater than ever before. Where will you stand my brothers when you hear the call?

Let's stand on the side of truth, integrity, peace and nobleness. Let's create our holistic health.

Rise up my Brothers, sing and be free!

I'm calling you out my noble brothers. Get tested for herpes. Treat your herpes. Warn your partners. Respect yourself. Be shining lights in this dark world. Let's all be Mandelas.

Part Two:

Sex and Love with Herpes

Chapter Eight:

The Ethics of a Life-Long Herpes Infection

From day one my own personal life-long herpes infection has presented me with several ethical challenges. It has challenged me on the question of who to tell and when. It has challenged me on the issue of what to say and how to say it. It has challenged me on the question of "Do I have any responsibilities towards trying to prevent the people in the community who do not have herpes from getting it, and if so what are they?"

On how to tell and when:

When I was diagnosed with herpes the doctors told me that it was safe to have sex with others as long as I avoided having sex during outbreaks and that I would get warning signs of when an outbreak would be coming. Luckily, we are working with much better information these days. A person with herpes is potentially contagious every-single day of the year and safer sex including using a combination of a condom and an anti-viral gel is the best way of ensuring that one isn't inadvertently spreading the virus.

I was an irresponsible coward when I first got herpes. Because the doctors told me that I wasn't contagious without outbreaks and because I was in the habit of using condoms, I decided that I only had to tell someone that I had herpes if and when it seemed like the relationship was turning serious and there would be regular sexual contact. I had justified my cowardice by thinking that the risk to others was too small to stick my neck out and get the rejection due to a herpes leper. Please don't be like me. Not telling someone before you have sex that you have herpes is absolutely the wrong thing to do. There's no real way to justify it. I now tell potential lovers I have herpes even before the first date. It gets the weight off my chest and feels like the right thing to do. (If you are a sex worker or are in the context of being in a sex club or party, there isn't the same disclosure obligation as in relationship in your personal life, but the imperative of safer sex is just as high if not higher)

Many people tell me that it's okay if you're not going to have sex with someone to wait and see if the relationship becomes serious before telling them about herpes. Sure this is much better than waiting until after sex, but to me it still isn't good enough. If you care about someone, if you respect them, why not tell them as early as possible so they can decide if they want to invest the energy and time in getting to know you better? Isn't it a bit manipulative to allow someone to develop feelings for you without warning them that they risk a life-long viral infection if they get involved with you?

Think about it, if you wait until they are already emotionally attached to you, they may feel compelled to continue with the relationship when they may not have if you had told them up-front. It takes more courage and integrity to tell early but it feels better to have the weight off your chest and the person you tell will usually respect you for giving them the choice.

I am especially reaching out to men, since I believe that men are not as protective as women of their sex partners when it comes to telling about herpes. Guys please don't have sex with anyone without telling them about your herpes. And if they don't know the facts, don't understate the risks; herpes is a more physically and emotionally devastating disease for

73

women than it is for men and it is much easier for a man to give a woman herpes than it is for a woman to give it to a man.

On how and what to say to others with herpes:

I am a holistic healer, an herbalist. My family has been healers for many generations in my native country of Trinidad and Tobago and in South America and as far back as Africa. I had little to no interest in treating herpes as a healer until I got herpes myself. Wanting to change a negative to a positive, I decided to make the holistic treatment of herpes the cornerstone of my practice. The bible says "the stone that the builder refused, I will make my cornerstone". Bob Marley and the wailers sing about it too.

It didn't take me long once I decided to become a holistic viral specialist to realize that I was confronted with a daunting challenge. Most professionals including all the herbalists and homeopaths I know rely heavily on referrals to build their client-base. Here I was now working with a client-base that I was never going to get a lot of referrals from.

My patients with herpes don't go around telling the world that I helped them with their outbreaks. Some of my patients have yet to tell their significant others that they have herpes, many have not told their closest friends and their family. I am not a company. I don't have an advertising budget. The only way for me to reach out to others with herpes and encourage them to come to me for treatment was to speak out in public about my herpes work and about herpes in general. This forced me to be far more out of the closet than would have been my personal choice.

I seem to always create challenging situations for myself. Speaking to others with herpes is not a task for the faint of heart. Some people like to shoot the messenger. I have the bullet-wounds to prove it. I can say that speaking to others with herpes has been, and continues to be, one of the most gratifying experiences in my life. I feel a deep bond with many of the people with herpes who interact with me. I felt this kind of bond when I played team sports. I've felt this kind of bond all my life with other black people. There's something about "us against the world" that can make people tight with each other. I love my herpes friends. I love my herpes patients; even the ones who misbehave. Nevertheless, the truth hurts, and I have some bitter truth to tell others with herpes.

Having a lover who also has herpes isn't a free ticket for unprotected sex. Even if you both have the same strain, even if one gave it to the other. Having unprotected sex with each other can make one or both partner's cases of herpes worse and you can infect each other in previously uninfected locations on your body. It's called inoculation and re-inoculation and it's a message many with herpes don't want to hear.

If you have herpes or cold sores you are potentially contagious everyday and there is no sure way to tell if you are shedding virus. So do consider using a condom/dental dam combined with an anti-viral gel when having sex and do be careful about sharing wet towels or wash cloths with others.

No two people get herpes the same way so you are going to have your own individual experience with the virus and will have to find your own way of dealing with it on all the different levels you will have to deal with it.

A cure for herpes in our lifetime is unlikely and there are no quick-fix solutions for managing herpes. Herpes cannot be managed with a topical agent alone; whether it is creams, lotions, or essential oils. Managing herpes takes changing your diet, managing stress and other triggers, and may also require either taking herbal medicine or drug therapy.

You may not get fewer outbreaks as you get older. While this is often the case, since no two people get herpes the same way, other diseases, menopause, self-abuse, re-inoculation by unprotected sex and other factors can change the pattern of frequency and severity of outbreaks at any point during your life-long journey with herpes.

Cold-sores are just as contagious if not more contagious than genital herpes and you can infect others when there are no signs of sores present.

Having herpes does make you more vulnerable to other sexually transmitted infections including HIV and HPV.

Daily use of l-lysine is an ineffective strategy for treating herpes and can do more harm than good. There are more effective natural remedies for herpes without side-effects.

On talking to those who don't have herpes:

The reality check for me is that the mainstream and alternative media do not want to talk about herpes. They would prefer to keep us in a ghetto. There is a lot of misinformation floating around and people without herpes have few places to turn to hear the facts about herpes. They don't hear the facts in their churches; young people are not being educated enough about herpes in school. Most parents aren't teaching their children about herpes, older siblings are not passing information down to the younger ones.

It's really up to us who have herpes to try harder to dialogue with those who don't.

It is my unshakable conviction that those of us in the herpes community need to be more vocal in the media and to also reach out to those around us. Each one teach one. Each one reach one.

Chapter Nine:

Love in a Time of Herpes

I was born in 1965, a year often considered the first year of "generation-x". The previous generation, the baby boomers like my parents, grew up in a time of free love. My mother didn't take advantage of this but my father sure did, but that's another story.

Us gen-x'ers were the first generation to have to deal with AIDS and the fallout from it. Instead of the sexual revolution we had fear and loathing in our own pants.

Now as a Holistic Herpes Treatment Specialist I treat a lot of teenagers and people in the early twenties who are exploring their sexuality in a time where we are no longer nearly as afraid of AIDS as we were in the eighties but where almost everyone has herpes. I often see girls as young as 15 who already have herpes and who got it from their first sexual experience. No one told them they could get herpes from fellatio. No one told them much of anything about sexually transmitted infections. It's a sad, sad thing to have to tell a teenager that they now have a life-long incurable disease and have to warn potential sex partners about it beforehand. This sentence drives many to the brink of despair. One 17 year old who got herpes from her first and only sex partner was crying hysterically on the phone with me, asking how in her small town of 1500 people can she tell anyone that she has herpes? She said she will not date or have sex again until she moves far away, and I believe her.

With oral sex being as common as hand-shakes used to be, why aren't we educating grade school students about sexually transmitted infections? Very few of the most at-risk population know that they can catch or pass on herpes when there are no signs of an outbreak. They don't know that they can get herpes on their genitals from contact with people who get cold sores on their mouth. They aren't empowered to say no way when they encounter sores and rashes and are told that "they are nothing".

Further exasperating the situation is the porn industry being a bad role model. Like myself and many of my generation, young people these days get a lot of their sex education from being exposed to porn. In the adult film industry condoms are almost never worn during oral sex and only worn during anal and oral sex about 40% of the time. I did three years of research into the adult film industry and learned that porn performers are tested monthly or more often for HIV but are rarely tested for herpes or HPV. Very few porn performers admit their herpes infections for fear of losing work and a backlash from their fans.

My older patients don't tend to fare much better than the younger ones. They don't know the facts about love in a time of herpes and most didn't do much to try and educate themselves. And for the ones that do try to educate themselves through the internet, they are confronted with a wilderness of websites saying many contradictory things, spreading a lot of misinformation and luring people with magical quick-fixes and snake oils. The message doesn't seem to be getting out to people that there are no quick-fixes for a life-long viral infection, that herpes cannot be managed with topical oils, or creams or liquids and that herbal medicine or drug therapy combined with proper diet, stress reduction and making peace with herpes are the only ways I have seen in my 16 years of experience to successfully manage herpes over the long-haul.

Because the fear of catching the HIV virus isn't what it used to be, too many people are becoming complacent about practicing safer sex. Many tell me they don't want to use condoms because of the lack of spontaneity. Many want the risk and pleasure of unprotected sex. I can relate to all of this, I don't particularly like condoms myself. But in this day and age it is not smart to have unprotected sex with someone you are not in a monogamous relationship with. Unless this is the case, do use a condom or anti-viral gel or better yet use them both together. Oral sex is sex and is risky sex so do practice safer sex with fellatio and cunnilingus as well.

Before the sex comes the sex-conversation. A conversation

many people never have before getting together. It is your right and responsibility to ask a potential sex partner what their history of sexually transmitted infections is, and use your best lie-detecting skills when listening. You must volunteer the same information yourself. Please do understand that most people have never had a real herpes test in their life. Regular STD testing panels do not test for herpes or genital warts. Swabbing is an unreliable way of testing for herpes. So unless your potential sex partner has had a recent type-specific serum blood test for herpes like the Western Blot test, they have no way of knowing if they have herpes or not and so then neither do you.

Unless someone has had a recent herpes test, I recommend that you assume that they have herpes and use a condom combined with an anti-viral prophylactic gel. Statistics show that anyone who has had more than two sex partners has a 20% chance of having herpes. More than four sex partners gives you a 40% chance of having herpes and more than 6 sex partners gives you a 60% chance of having herpes. And of course herpes is only one of many sexually transmitted infections a person could have.

If anyone is elusive or sketchy about wanting to discuss their sexual health it's best to assume that they have something they are trying to hide. I don't mean to sound harsh or cynical; I'm an idealist by nature. I have listened to too many of my patients grieving over the fact that they were deceived by the person who infected them with herpes. You lose nothing by being careful and looking out for your own best interests.

(Email me at christopher.scipio@gmail.com if you'd like to learn more about how to have "the talk" with a potential lover)

I know it's a bummer but this is the reality of love and sex in a time of herpes. Love and love abundantly, but please be careful out there.

Overcoming Touch Deprivation.

From the time you were a newborn the amount of loving touch you received directly effected how well you thrived.

I was born two months premature in Trinidad in 1965. I weighed only 4 pounds and had to remain in an incubator for my first few weeks of life. The doctors told my mom not to get attached to me because I only had a ten percent chance of surviving. My mother didn't believe them. She touched and loved me and willed me to live. And live I did. I grew into being a 6'3", 200 pound man in almost perfect health. Such is the power of love, such is the power of touch.

We tend to get touched less and less as we get older, although our primal need for touch never diminishes. Touch deprivation is a significant form of sensory deprivation. Most of us wouldn't dream of going weeks or months without opening our eyes, or keeping our ears plugged, yet many of my patients tell me that they haven't been massaged or held for months or years.

Our world is becoming too formal, too stiff, too emotionally cold.

For the sake of your physical, emotionally, mental and spiritual health, give your self more permission to touch and be touched. You can never overdose on loving touch.

Don't limit touch to sex. Don't limit touch to just your partner and family. Reach out and touch more people. Close your eyes sometimes and experience your world through touch. Your skin is your biggest organ- use it. Get more skin to skin contact. Everyone can heal and be healed through touch. Be a great healer and lover by experiencing the miracle of touch as often as you can.

Chapter Ten:

How to Deal with Herpes Rejection

He or She Just Ain't That Into You.

If you have herpes and have the integrity to tell someone about it before you get sexually involved and they reject you because of it, it is one of the most devastating forms of rejection imaginable. Just as bad as being rejected because of your race, or physical disability or anything else not under your control, and just as ignorant and intolerable.

When the people I treat tell me their rejection stories I feel for them. Some are so shaken by it that they stop dating for years or ghettoize themselves to only dating others with herpes.

What I say to them is that "He or She was just not that into You". No one who really wants a person, and I do mean want the person, the whole person and the package that comes with them, will reject them just because they have herpes. Who would want that kind of superficial love anyways?

Herpes is a great litmus test to let you know who really cares about you and desires you.

It's reasonable for someone to want the risks and consequences explained to them. It's reasonable for someone not to be enthusiastic about you having herpes. Who would be? But anyone who really loved you or thought you were sexy before finding out about your herpes will still think so afterwards.

When you further explain to them that you are managing your herpes with herbal medicine or drug therapy and that you practice safer sex with a condom and an anti-viral gel there should be no reason for them not to want to sex you up right then and there.

Hold your head up high. Remember who you are; how special you are; how deserving you are of love and all its fruits. Don't let anyone diss you or make you feel less than. Anyone who wants you must accept the whole package of your life. Don't settle for anything less than that.

Chapter 11:

A Safer Sex Primer for the Herpes Nation

Have Sex:

A happy and life-affirming sex life is your God/dess given right. Don't feel that you have to opt out of the joys of life just because you have a life-long herpes infection. It's not easy to feel sexy when you are having regular outbreaks, especially if you are a woman, but it's important to feel like a whole, clean, desirable person.

I've written before and I'll write it again: having herpes doesn't make you any less attractive or sexy or moral or clean as you were before you got herpes. Perception can be very deceptive, especially the way many people choose to see themselves. You have the power to change how you see yourself for the better. If you want sex and are not having any symptoms of an outbreak or prodrome there's no reason in the world not to have sex. Beyond the physical pleasures, intimacy is vital in this all too cold world.

Have sex but be responsible with your sexuality.

Whether or not to have Safer Sex:

In my opinion, it is the right and responsibility of any two or more consenting adults about to start a sexual relationship, even if it's a casual one, to have a conversation about whether or not they wish to practice safer sex. I encourage people to have safer sex but no one has the right to tell anyone what to do with their own body. Some people like taking risks; some are down-right self-destructive and destructive to others.

Some choose to smoke cigarettes or do recreational drugs. Some eat junk food. Some watch junk tv.

Whatever the two or more people about to begin a sexual relationship decide, it should be a mutual agreement. Don't leave it to assumptions or reading between the lines. Don't have your head in the sand. Don't fantasize that God or Spirit or good luck is a substitute for a safer sex strategy. Talk about it openly and decide what level of risk is appropriate for the situation.

Know Your Partner: Get Tested

Having sex with any person who hasn't recently been tested for sexually transmitted infections including having blood tests for herpes, hepatitis, and HPV is like playing Russian roulette. Not only would you not know what you may be exposing yourself to, but the person in question may be in the dark themselves. Some people would rather not know than know.

Don't be intimidated to ask. In this day in age it isn't disloyal or rude or unromantic to ask about someone's sexually transmitted infection status.

If you do not know your partner's test status it's best to assume that they have at least one sexually transmitted infection and to govern yourself accordingly. If you do not know your test results you should also assume that you have at least one sexually transmitted infection and should take the appropriate precautions to inform and protect your partner/s.

Know Your Limits: Stick to Your Comfort Zone:

A lot of people, especially women, get intimidated by their partners into engaging in sexual acts that are outside of their comfort zone. Do not allow anyone to pressure you into doing anything you are not ready, willing and able to do. It's your body, exercise the fullness of your rights.

It's all a matter of choice. No one is less cool or less committed to any relationship by sticking to their own sexual boundaries.

Use a Condom or Barrier:

Safer sex means using a condom for genital, oral and anal sex if there is a penis involved or a dental dam or saran wrap if there isn't a penis involved. If someone is allergic to latex there are polyurethane condoms available. For oral sex there are flavoured condoms as an option.

Please don't use a condom that contains a spermicide as these tend to irritate your mucous membranes and make the people involved more likely to get a sexually transmitted infection.

Don't develop a false sense of security with condoms/dental dams/saran wrap. These do not cover areas of the body that can still transmit and be vulnerable to infection. Using an antiviral gel on possible transmission and infection sites can help lessen this possibility. For example, if a man gets herpes sores in his pubic hair area or perineum or buttocks, wearing a condom will not protect his partner; using an antiviral gel may.

Condoms can also break or slip off. Using an anti-viral gel underneath a condom will help protect in the case of a broken or slipped-off condom. Using a water-based lube or anti-viral gel outside of the condom will reduce the likelihood of the condom breaking.

The condom should go on as soon as the clothes come off if not before.

Once a man has ejaculated, he should remove the condom from his penis and remove his penis from intimate contact with his partner as condoms are very likely to slip off as the penis becomes flaccid.

If you are practicing fisting, latex gloves are recommended.

Use an Antiviral Gel:

I have been treating herpes holistically for 25 years now, starting with my own. Even during the heady days twelve years ago when I finally was able to put together an effective protocol for controlling herpes outbreaks, I was still left with a daunting challenge.

Yes, now I knew I could greatly limit the frequency and severity of outbreaks with the virus for myself and others, in fact I could keep many people outbreak free for vast stretches of time, but that still wasn't enough of a safeguard against infecting others with this lifelong viral illness.

The fear of passing herpes on to loved ones kept myself and keeps many others reluctant to have a sex life at all, and ironically, having a happy and active sex life is one of the best ways to keep the virus dormant. Happy, sexually active people are less likely to have outbreaks.

Condoms are of course a great tool in making sex safer. But there are problems with condoms, they can break or slide off. They don't offer much help if the man's site for herpes or genital warts are in locations other than the penis, i.e. buttocks, legs, etc.

The Bill and Melinda Gates Foundation spent twenty-five million dollars researching natural microbiocides to find natural barriers that would protect women in the third world from HIV. What they discovered is that Carrageenan, a natural component of some red and brown seaweeds, is an effective barrier which inhibits the ability of HPV, herpes and other STIs (Sexually Transmitted Infections) from replicating on the surface of the skin and inhibits their ability to adhere to the skin. I developed my own microbiocide with Carrageenan and other substances. My microbiocide (Anti-Viral Gel) is edible, completely non-toxic and can act as a lubricant. It is not meant as a replacement for condoms, it's designed as a supplement to condom use to make it less likely to infect your loved ones. It's effective for genital, anal and oral sex.

You use the gel as a barrier so the best way to use it in terms of heterosexual sex is for the man to put some on his penis and then put a latex condom on the penis. Then a small amount of gel would be applied to the labia of the woman and also inside her vagina. The gel should be reapplied every 30-45 minutes. Even after being sucked or licked there is enough of a coating of the gel to be effective for 30 minutes. The gel can be used as a barrier in anal sex, oral sex, lesbian oral sex and even for kissing.

The gel should be used with a latex condom or a dental dam/

saran wrap. The gel is not a contraceptive and will not prevent pregnancy.

To inquire about ordering the gel email me or visit http://www.antiviralgel.com

Urinate After Sex:

It is crucially important for women to urinate as soon after sex as possible. I recommend that it be within 15 minutes of completing the act. Failing to do so on a regular basis can lead to urinary tract and bladder infections.

I recommend that men follow this advice as well.

Do You Dare to be Outbreak Free?

It has been said that often what you get in life is what you expect to get. This is the root cause of why, for example, so many people who are born in poverty die in poverty, or why someone who has failed several times to quit a bad habit has a hard time believing that he or she can succeed the next time. Certainly the past doesn't equal the future - sounds reasonable enough on paper. But whom am I trying to kid? We are emotional creatures and logic often cannot stand a challenge from deeply embedded feelings.

I see this challenge affecting many of my herpes patients and it affected me for many years too. In the film "The Shawshank Redemption" there was an older prisoner who had been in jail his whole life. When he was finally paroled he was petrified of the outside world and even tried to get himself re-admitted to prison. Finally he hung himself. The character played by Tim Robbins asked why this happened and Morgan Freeman's character replied that it was "institutionalized."

Anytime you get used to a certain series of events occurring whether it is the daily routine of prison or regular herpes outbreaks, your mind becomes convinced of the certainty of those events repeating themselves. One of the hardest things to do in the world of human behaviour is to break the pattern of these expectations. It takes a lot of imagination and daring.

To be free of outbreaks one has to believe in a future without outbreaks. One has to see it, feel it, and believe it. It has to be an unshakeable conviction because your mind knows when you are just going through the motions.

It's hard to be convinced that outbreaks don't have to be part of the experience of a life-long herpes infection, but it's not impossible.

One approach that I know can work is what I call "incrementalism" or taking "baby-steps". You may not be able to get to your goal in giant strides, but you can get there one tiny step at a time. If you are having outbreaks every month, if you can manage to go one month without an outbreak, that is a step in the right direction and a confidence builder, then make a two month reprieve from outbreaks happen, then try for three. Even if you have an outbreak after two or three months, don't despair, you are making progress and you can build on this. If you persist and don't fall into despair with a set-back, soon you will be going longer and longer periods of time without outbreaks.

In manifesting a different future for yourself it's important to have the full support of your lover. One of the biggest obstacles to imagining an outbreak free future is the fear of giving herpes to your partner. Please do treat your herpes and please do practice safer sex with a condom/dental dam and an anti-viral gel. This will ease your mind, but it's not enough. I stopped having outbreaks when my girlfriend at the time told me that she wasn't afraid of getting herpes from me. This powerful declaration set me free.

I was no longer anxious when we were having sex. I never had an outbreak in the time we were together and have only had three in the past seven years, with only one in the past four years despite having a very busy and demanding holistic viral practice which often leaves me with no sleep and little time to eat on a regular schedule. If you have a partner who is very nervous about getting herpes from you, you may want to consider getting another partner or finding a way of addressing your partner's fears because the anxiety from a fearful partner coupled with your own fear of infecting an uninfected person, will often be enough to keep the cycle of outbreaks happening.

The last piece of advice I have to offer in this note is to stop seeing yourself as a victim. You are a human being. You have power. Use your power. You can reprogram your mind. You can change your expectations. You can make a peaceful accommodation with the herpes virus and ask it to stay dormant. You can holistically manage your herpes with diet, holistic stress management and herbal medicine or drug therapy. You can practice safer sex to protect your lover/s and yourself.

In fact you can do almost anything you believe you can. What a human being can do is almost unlimited. What most people choose to do is disappointing. Choose differently. Dare to live outbreak free.

Chapter 12:

My Natropractica Holistic Herpes Protocol

Real Herbal Medicine and Why You Should Get Yours from an Herbalist

We need plants, they don't need us. They give us oxygen, building materials, food and medicine. We give them little except disrespect and destruction. They would be better off if we were not around. They will still be here long after we are no longer around.

Plants are living, evolving, complex life forms. They are not just a package of chemicals for our exploitation as scientists would like us to believe. They are the true masters of chemistry and can produce medicines far past our ability to even conceive.

When we turn to plants for healing, the energy and vitality of the plant/s in the plant medicine is just as important if not more so than the chemicals we wish to extract. Failing to even acknowledge the energetics of herbal medicine is one of the many failures of the cold, superficial approach of the drug companies. It's no wonder that plant medicine produces so few side-effects and virtually no deaths while synthetic drugs kills hundreds of thousands of people annually, and I'm not speaking of deaths from improper use. This is the number of people killed by proper use of pharmaceutical drugs.

When you buy so-called herbal medicine or natural medicine from the internet or health food stores or wherever, you are likely buying products brutally mass-produced on industrial machines that are the equivalent of the Kraft Dinners of plant medicine. You are receiving an impersonally made product rather than a medicine made by a professional medicine-maker. Herbal medicine has always been made and should be made either by an herbalist or by yourself. When you take the healer out of the medicine-making process you de-humanize the medicine. You end up getting cold, sterile, dead products made with the same manufacturing processes as a pharmaceutical drug with the same mentality as a pharmaceutical drug, namely to make a product with the least amount of expense, that is sterile and uniform, has no relationship to nature and that maximizes the companies' profit.

If you want a product that in no way tastes like, smells like, looks like or feels like the plants it came from and likely has had its molecules re-arranged to protect the companies' position in the marketplace, go ahead, but don't fool yourself into believing that you are taking real herbal medicine.

Is your herbal medicine in a liquid form? We evolved from the sea, as did all life on this planet. Your body is more than 80% liquid. The planet is 70% liquid. Plants are mostly liquid. Real herbal medicine is liquid. The tradition for the past 30,000 years or more is to make herbal medicine in the form of teas, decoctions and tinctures. The reason for this is that these forms preserve the energy and chemistry of the plants the best and liquid medicine, like liquid foods, are the easiest things for your body to assimilate. If you prefer capsules or pills to liquid remedies it's because you don't have enough respect for the plants you are turning to for help to be willing to experience their taste, aroma and energy. In that case maybe your should stick to those little coloured pills from the drug companies.

Do you know who made your herbal medicine? Who made your medicine and how it was made is just, if not more important, than what is in the medicine. For the best in plant medicine your medicine should be made by an herbalist or by you. Someone who will make your medicine with integrity and with the right thoughts and intentions. Someone who will only use healthy, ethically harvested plants. Someone who will not compromise on quality to make more money. Do you know where your medicine was made and what kind of energy it absorbed while being made?

When you take your herbal medicine can you feel, smell, taste or see anything of the plant/s used to make that medicine?

Does the medicine make you feel more connected to the plants when you put it into your body? Does it make you feel connected to the person who made it? Does it make you feel more connected in general?

Unless you can answer yes to all of the above questions, you are not taking real herbal medicine. Herbal medicine has been the main healing modality for human beings since the beginning and even today it continues to be the main source of medicine for 70% of the world's population. More and more people in the richest countries of the world are rejecting pharmaceutical drugs and their dangerous side-effects and returning to herbal medicine. If you wish to get the best that plant medicine has to offer, get your herbal medicine from an herbalist or learn how to make it yourself.

The Natural Health Products Hustle

False Prophets Chasing Profits

There was a time not too long ago when going to the health food store was a cherished adventure of mine. Back in the 70's and 80's when I was a kid, the health food store was this lone tiny outpost in the community where the owner was most certainly a holdout from Woodstock or some prophet crying out in the materialistic wilderness for us all to repent and find our way back to nature. It was really cool for me to go there and gawk at the Hippies, and Hare Krishnas and other "freaks" that would hang out there. I'd smell the patchouli and take in the funky hemp clothing and see the vast array of Birkenstocks.

The health food store was like a portal to an entirely other dimension. The products were usually in bulk bins or in plain wrapper or with nondescript labels. There was a minimum of packaging and processing. The natural remedies smelt, tasted and often even looked like the sources where they came from. The cheaply printed, usually self-published books were humble and sincere in a way that seems strangely quaint now and the owner spoke softly and patiently but with the passion of an evangelist.

Like Stevie Wonder says "I wish those days, would come back once more, I wish those days, never had to go, I loved them so."

It's been a long time since going to a health food store was regarded as a fringe activity. Now there are health food stores in the smallest of communities and there are even several big chains of health food stores that are far swankier than most mainstream grocery stores.

You have to have a pretty good income to shop in many of the heath food stores I've been to lately. But I guess it's all a sign of positive progress. People are more interested in health foods and natural remedies than they have been in a long time.

The biggest change has been in the natural remedies. There are now scores of companies making innumerable brands of supplements and remedies. It's a huge business now, virtually a gold rush, and lots of people have rushed right into the market. Many of the old time supplement companies have been bought by food companies like Kraft and by pharmaceutical companies.

The packaging is slick; the form of the "natural remedies" is often so sterile and processed that there is little resemblance to the plants and natural materials they were extracted from.

Everyday it seems, doctors and scientists point out that many of these "natural" products and remedies are either dangerous or have no therapeutic value, and in many cases I would have to agree with them.

Once again, though, nature is not to blame.The natural world produces the most powerful and effective healing substances ever known. Natural medicine, like natural living, restores our vitality and grace in ways synthetic medicine cannot begin to touch.

What is to blame is simply greed and human arrogance. I'll deal with the greed first.

With the natural health products gold rush has come a gold rush mentality. Often when vitamins and supplements and other natural products were independently tested, it has been discovered that they either didn't contain the medicinal ingredient promised or they contained it in much smaller quantities than stated.

Back in the day, natural health products companies were pioneers, mavericks and in my opinion, heroes. They weren't there just for the money; frankly there wasn't that much money to be made. They were promoting an alternative to our love affair with chemicals and self-pollution. Now it seems that I can't go anywhere without being bombarded with outrageous claims and dodgy marketing practices both in and off the internet. They have people, including myself at times, running from here to there bewildered by what one is really supposed to be taking for one's health. The sad fact is that some of this misinformation out there has granted governments all around the world the excuse to start cracking down on natural health products. Here in Canada they have even gone to the extent of banning Comfrey, although I don't see how they believe they can ban something that grows in most people's gardens.

The timing couldn't be worse. The population is more dependent on prescription drugs than ever before and more people are dying or being harmed from the use of prescription drugs than ever before. Added to that is the sad reality that many people are also suffering from environmental and cultural pollution.

The other component to the natural health products hustle is arrogance.

Nature has been producing amazing medicinals for billions of years. We have recently shown up on this planet with our oversized brains and undersized understanding, and after what hasn't even been a cosmic blink of the eye we have decided that we can do better than nature. We have decided that we can standardize nature.

Standardization doesn't exist in nature; in fact it's against the laws of nature. Nature revolves around diversity. It's the law of variation. Populations, whether they be plant or animal, with a good variation of genes are healthy and populations without are inbred. No two snowflakes are the same, no two plants are alike. That's the way it's meant to be. But of course that wasn't good enough for some of the natural health products companies. They decided that it was better to artificially manipulate and process nature to suit their own designs. After the gold rush started, an arm's race started over standardizing vitamins and supplements and remedies. Companies began to experiment with ways to extract more of certain identified compounds out of plants and minerals. In doing so they created their own arms race with different companies competing to see who could build the best natural health products Frankenstein's monster. Their approach isn't fundamentally different than the pharmaceutical companies'. It's the same shit just different pills.

We don't standardize wine. Can you imagine if we made it so that every year the Chablis from all over the world tasted the same and had the exact same chemical signature?

It's a bit of a mockery that in the same health food stores where people are being encouraged to return to eating unprocessed organic fruits and vegetables there are shelve loads of natural health products that don't smell, look or taste like the plants and minerals they come from, produced by high-tech extraction and processing methods. These natural health products are the equivalent of eating at McDonald's or having a TV dinner.

Some will always prefer synthetic to natural, man-made to organic. Not all these products are bad, not all of these products are unhelpful. It's the state of consciousness behind them that concerns me the most. Instead of investing the time and money to more fully investigate the natural medicines all around us, these arrogant greedy companies prefer to remake nature in their own images.

Despite the fact that most of the world is water and that most of our bodies are liquid, they have fallen in love all over again with the pill and here we go living in the "Valley of the Dolls".

Like the holdout owners of those health food stores back in the day, I am here to speak out to anyone that will listen. If we believe in the adage from Hippocrates "Let medicine be thy food and thy food be thy medicine," then let's treat medicine like food and keep it as natural and organic as possible, without the unnecessary intervention of technology. Let's keep all the diversity and variance that nature has designed. Let's use whole botanical and other extracts instead of isolating single compounds like the drug companies do.

I don't have any suggestions on how to compel these companies from marketing snake oil to the public. I do however have some suggestions on how individuals can empower themselves in this precarious environment.

1. Don't Put Your Faith in False Gods.

Don't put your faith in pills or associations or initials after someone's name, or in white lab coats or government decrees or rumours or advertising or peer pressure or even in what I have to say.

Use your own judgment. Use your intuition, challenge all premises and go within. Your own body is the Great Healer, Nature is the Great Medicine. Look around you, there's medicine all around you. Go to the source. Use medicines in the simplest, most natural forms possible. Don't look for packaging, look for healing power. Don't let anyone or anything intimidate you. You have the intelligence and intuition to learn about natural healing.

2. Don't Be Lazy.

Health isn't something you can go to a store or an office and buy. Health is a state of consciousness and a lifestyle. In many ways health is a state of grace. Unless you are living in the state of grace of being in harmony with yourself, your relationships and your environment, then you cannot experience full holistic health.

3. Embrace Real Healers.

There is healing energy everywhere. In a loving mother nursing her child. In lovemaking on its deepest levels, in a crowd's euphoria over their team's victory, in dancing to music that resonates with your soul.

You know what that energy feels like, so when you go to see a naturopath or homeopath or traditional healer or physician or minister or Reiki practitioner, any healer whatsoever, if you don't feel that loving/healing energy from them, if you don't feel that they deeply care about you, move on! You won't find true healing without the true healing energy.

But when you do find a true healer, embrace them. Embrace the magic and respect the healing.

4. Make Your Own Medicines

Never making your own remedies is like never cooking for yourself. No meal is better than one prepared with love. And whenever someone cooks with love they think about the love they share for the people the food is intended for and that love finds its way into the food. And that loving cook is going to be very selective about the ingredients that go into that meal and that loving discrimination finds itself into the meal, and so it is with making your own remedies.

If you never made your own tinctures I encourage you to do so. If you don't know how to, email me and I'll send you directions on how to do it. It's inexpensive, it's fun, it's empowering. There's no downside whatsoever, so do go out and experience the joy of making natural remedies. Your body will feel the difference too.

Why I Love Making My Own Remedies

I come from a long line of Afro-Caribbean herbalists and bush doctors. I was born in Trinidad and was first exposed to natural healing by my maternal grandmother who was a well-respected healer. My grandmother was quite a character. 101

She wore a white turban and used a crystal ball. She put herself and others into trances and communicated with the spirit world. She would go into the rain forests of Trinidad to wildcraft plants for her bush baths, teas and medicines. Everything she made she made in her kitchen or in the backyard. It was wonderful seeing sick people who the doctors had sent away to die get healed.

Both my great-grandmothers on my mother's side were Carib Indian medicine women in Guyana, South America.

From the age of 18 on I used massage and herbal remedies to heal myself and my friends and the people around me, but I had no intention of becoming a practitioner since I was consumed with my photography and film directing careers, but life stepped in and changed my path. I was almost killed in a car accident. What horrified me the most was not the accident or the injuries it left me with, but rather it was the treatment (actually, mistreatment) I received from the emergency room staff and the doctors who dealt with me. It made me realize how many other people out there were suffering from the poor care and drugs they were receiving from western medicine. I decided to become a full time healer and do what I could to help as many as I could. It was not easy to switch to being a part-time artist after 18 years but I did it nonetheless. So here I am a full time holistic viral specialist and herbalist based in Canada, but I never forgot what I learned from my grandmother and the most important thing she taught me was to make my own medicines. In healing, everything is part of the equation. Who the healer is is a huge factor. You bring everything that you are, everything you have ever done, everywhere you have ever been, everything you have ever touched on any level to the healing.

If you cannot come as a healer with clean hands, clean energy and a clean heart, you contaminate the healing. How the remedies are made and where the materials come from are also crucial factors.

I already live in an impersonal, automated, mass-produced culture. Do I want the medicines I am giving to people to be machine-made, impersonally mass-produced, with materials which I have no idea where they came from, what condition they were in and who grew or collected them? The answer for me is… not if I can help it! I can't make every remedy that I use, some things are just too hard to get right now, but I am determined to make everything that I can. I make my herbal medicines in a more expensive and time consuming way than the norm but have no regrets doing so because you can tell the difference in the finished product. I was gathering "seaweeds" at the beach last week and many people came up to me to ask what I was doing. They were very puzzled at seeing me spend so much time and energy gathering things they hadn't given a second thought to. It struck me that we, including myself, are so oblivious sometimes to the medicines all around us. I think back to the countless times I have been in beaches and forests and other wild places and didn't see the medicines. I think of how we whacked and kicked dandelions when I was a kid growing up in Toronto. I think of the 1400 or so species of medicinal plants that go extinct every year in the Amazon basin alone.

If it sounds like I'm completely against science and technology, I'm not. I don't believe that there is any natural conflict between science and magic or between technology and art. As a photographer I learned that if you are too fixated on the technical you will never be able to develop your vision and will never create art. And if you ignore the technical aspects you will never have mastery over your craft.

I make my remedies with the technical aspects in mind. I use dry-weights, solubility factors, specific gravity, acidity and other technical factors to inform how I make remedies. But never to the exclusion of the magic and emotional relationship between myself and the substances. I spend a lot of time and focus and a lot of energy on the remedies. I think about who they are for and what ailments they are meant to address. I think about where they came from and who they came from. I synchronize the making of the remedies to the cycles of the moon and get a lot of excitement watching the remedies develop. I greatly enjoy the different colours and textures and aromas. It can be a very sensual experience. I have promised myself to no longer be swayed by packaging and brand names. I want to know where my medicines come from, who made them and how much healing energy they have before I use them with my clients and loved ones. As a Healer I want to keep my medicines as raw and natural as possible. I think my grandmother would have been proud.

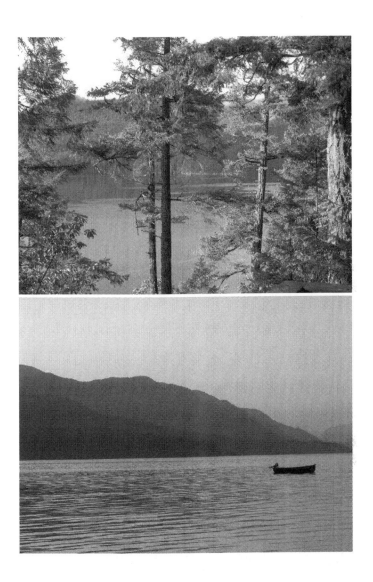

How My Remedies Are Made

In May of 2003 I completed the move (after a six month stop in Vancouver) from the Upper Westside of Manhattan to a small coastal community of 6000 people in British Columbia,

Canada, accessible only by boat or plane. As you can see from the photos above of my neighbourhood, this coastal community is surrounded by a pristine temperate rain forest which is one of the richest varieties of medicinal plants anywhere in the world. We are blessed with the world's best "seaweeds" and mosses and lichens, and the moderate climate allows many land-based plants to grow all year round. One of my friends even has a banana plant thriving in her garden. We have also just been blessed with one of the best medicinal mushroom seasons in recent memory with Reishis and Turkey Tails and Chanterelles and many other species popping out everywhere including my own driveway.

I miss living in New York City but being here in the bush surrounded by this magnificent nature and tranquility has profoundly changed both me and my healing practice forever. I now spend most of my time foraging in the woods and beaches for plants, raiding my friends' and neighbours' organic herb gardens and making remedies in my lab. I can't describe how much I'm enjoying all of this.

The bottom line is that I now make 90% of my remedies myself from scratch. I am working with happy, healthy plants picked at the optimal time of their growing cycle. I am using pure, Canadian Artesian spring water for my water-based remedies and Jamaican Overproof rum as my favourite menstruum for my tinctures. I am slow cooking for days the remedies on a wood stove over Douglas Fir and Alder wood in traditional clay pots. I am making the remedies the old fashioned way like my grandmother and probably your grandmother did. The remedies are prepared by hand; most are never touched by a machine. The only machine I own is a blender.

From the time I obtain the plant to the time it leaves for the post office, my hands are the only hands that have touched your remedy. This continuity of Intent and Attention is vitally important.

Although they are still so far behind what Holistic Healers have known for eons, the scientists are starting to catch up. The current understanding of quantum physics states that the presence of an observer has a profound and measurable effect on the object being observed. It has been demonstrated that an object can behave like a wave when no one is looking and then revert to behaving like a particle in the presence of an observer. It has been stated in quantum physics that an object can appear simultaneously in many positions when not being observed but will immediate assume one position in the presence of an observer. It has been proven by experiments that water crystals will change shape to mimic words or thoughts in their vicinity. I won't get into the merits of quantum physics but if you are interested or skeptical do look into it yourself or watch the film "What the Bleep Do We Know?" or go to http://www.whatthebleep.com.

What I will point out is that if the presence of a casual observer can have a powerful effect on the objects around them, imagine what the effect of a healer's intent and attention can have on remedies and the healing of a patient?

Who makes your remedies, and their intent and focus, is just as important, if not more so than what's in a remedy. When I make my remedies I focus on the person the remedy is for and for the ailment it's meant to heal. I have seen over and over again the difference in receiving a remedy from a healer versus buying one off the shelf in which you have had no interaction with the persons who made the medicine, have no idea where the medicine was made, what condition the ingredients were in, how the medicine was prepared and the intent involved.

As I pointed out before, the planet is 70% water and your body is over 80% water. To me it's vitally important to receive your medicine in liquid form whenever possible. Not only is it the most natural way for your body to absorb medicine but water has superior abilities to carry the energy signature of the plant the medicine was made from.

Moving Away from a Dependence on Substance-based Medicine

One of the few things upon which Natural healers and scientists agree is that the universe is energetic rather than material-based.

Yet both allopathic and much of Natural Medicine still place a heavy emphasis on healing through taking substances.

Taking substances can be a powerful component of a healing plan. In the case of Natural medicine the remedies can re-connect us with the natural world and allow us to harness the billions of years of experience of the plant master chemists. But I caution you not to focus too much on substances when you have so much healing power within you.

Love is the ultimate engine of healing. Love is unlimited, inexhaustible, transcendent, illuminating, liberating.

Liberation is key. Often our chronic illnesses are a result of our failure to break free of negative patterns of thoughts, feelings and behaviours. Love can change anything. Love can set you free.

Without an abundance of love, healing will never be complete.

If and when you take a substance to aide your healing, spend at least five minutes focusing and directing your mind/spirit on what you want the medicine to do for your healing. Feel the medicine's effect on your body, and pay close attention to how your body reacts. If you cannot do this at first keep trying until you can.

You have the power to become a healing alchemist. You can transform the substances you take into your body into the healing instrument that you need. You can limit the negative side-effects of prescription drugs with your personal power. You can make natural medicines more effective.

You can even turn water into wine. So unlimited is your potential.

Herpes and the Therapeutic Importance of Sleep

We live in a macho culture where even women and children brag about how little sleep they can get by with, as if depriving oneself of sleep is an Olympic feat. I actually consider the opposite to be true. I consider depriving oneself of sleep as a form of self-abuse. Policemen, intelligence officers and army interrogators from Gitmo to Syria, Zimbabwei and many local police stations know that depriving prisoners of sleep is one the most effective techniques in forcing "co-operation".

To be holistically healthy almost everyone needs between 7 to 8.5 hours of quality sleep each day- this is especially important for those of us with herpes. Sleep deprivation is a common trigger for severe herpes outbreaks. If you cannot get that much sleep at night you should make up for it with a long nap or extra sleep on your days off- contrary to popular myth, naps that are 90 minutes or longer are far more beneficial than "cat naps." The best time of the day to nap is the afternoon, hence the age old tradition of the siesta.

In as few as 4 days in a row of less than 7 hours of quality sleep we dramatically start to lose our ability to make sound decisions, start having short-term memory problems and we even start to become pre-diabetic. If you continue to be sleep deprived you will quickly start displaying dysfunctional even psychotic behaviour.

Sleep-deprived people are far more likely to be angry, violent, irritable and irrational. Brain scans show the brains of sleep-deprived people behave similarly to those with the most serious mental health issues. If you oversleep you will be far more prone to depression so the key is to get the right amount of quality sleep.

When you are feeling ill, even if it's simply a cold or flu coming on- the most important thing is to call in sick, clear your schedule and get plenty of sleep and bed-rest, this is essential for dealing with herpes outbreaks as well.

For men sleep-deprivation will diminish your ability to perform sexually. For both men and women lack of sleep with reduce your fertility.

And for the vain ones reading this missive, lack of sleep most definitely will reduce your beauty.

Not only is getting 7-8.5 hours of quality sleep important but it is essential that we get enough "deep-sleep" because even if you are in bed for the required amount of time but are woken up or disturbed enough you will not get enough "deep-sleep". The older you are the more important "deep-sleep" is. A person in their 30's gets 100 minutes of deep sleep each night, by the time you are in your 60's you only get 20 minutes of "deep-sleep".

Without enough "deep-sleep" you can develop diabetes, high blood pressure, heart disease, stroke and many other health problems. "Deep-sleep" is important for your immune system and for keeping the herpes virus dormant.

To ensure you get the "deep-sleep" you need: Don't drink or eat anything within 2 hours of bedtime- eating before sleep can give you bad dreams and drinking may force you to wake up to go to the bathroom. Make sure you sleep in an environment that is dark, quiet and comfortable- wear ear plugs and/or a blindfold if needed. Don't allow children or pets to wake you up if you can avoid it. Don't allow someone else's snoring to wake you up if you can avoid it.

Don't watch the news, music videos, or disturbing imagery just before going to bed. If you are wound up have a hot bath, ask your partner for a massage or have some sex or all of the above before going to bed. If you've had a fight with a loved one try to make peace before going to bed.

If you are studying or working on a deadline- it's been clinically proven that you get better results when you get a good night's sleep than to do an all-nighter or pushing yourself when you are exhausted.

There is a great many reasons why all animals sleep. Lack of sleep now guarantees negative health consequences in the future. I wish you all a lifetime of lovely, restorative, holistically healthy sleep.

The New Holistic Herpes Diet

Do's (Everyday unless otherwise noted)

Plain Organic Yoghurt (at least 2.5% milk fat)
Salmon or Sardines or Mackerel (at least 3-4 times per week)
Avocado
Extra Virgin Olive Oil
Blueberries, Strawberries, Blackberries
Other Fruit
Hemp Seeds, not Hemp Protein, 2-4 tablespoons
Flax Seeds
Chia Seeds
At least One Salad per day. (Avoid Salad Dressing You don't make Yourself.
Have Extra Virgin Olive Oil as the base for your Salad Dressing).
Make at least one smoothie a day with Kale or other Greens, Fruit, Yoghurt, Hemp Seeds, Avocado, etc
Tuna (once per week only)
Beans
Vegetables
Chicken or Poultry (only a few times a week at the most)
Eggs
Cheese (only a few times per week)
Kombucha tea, only if you make it yourself and make it without caffeine
Sauerkraut, Kim Chee and other fermented foods
Nutritional Yeast
Soup (at least once per day

Don'ts (Never)

Artificial Sweeteners
Sugar
Coffee, Green Tea, Black Tea, Cola Drinks, Chocolate
Nuts
Sesame Seeds, including Tahini
Poppy Seeds, Pumpkin Seeds, Sunflower Seeds
Dates, Carob, Raisins
Fruit Juices
Sodas
Cereal, Cereal Grains
Oatmeal
Bacon, Cold Cuts, Prepared Meats, Sausages
Beef
White Wine

Notes:

Reduce your intake of wheat, rice and flour as much as possible. Limiting to only few times a week if ever. Stay away from breads and pastas and bake goods including cakes and muffins and cookies and bagels. Its okay to have brown or wild rice, or whole grain quinoa a few times a week.

Limit your intake or Potatoes and other Starchy Vegetables such as Yams, and Sweet Potatoes to a few times a week at the most.

Try to reduce alcohol intake as much as possible.

Lifestyle and State of Consciousness:

The virus is going to be in your body for life, and believe it or not, it greatly prefers to stay dormant, much like its cousin the chicken-pox virus that is also a member of the herpes family of viruses and also in your body for life.

1. Forgive the person who gave you herpes. Even if you were deceived and put at risk without your consent, holding on to the anger and resentment not only aggravates your health but it also binds your psychologically to a negative event which you are powerless to change.

2. Forgive yourself for having herpes. Many people with herpes feel dirty, ashamed, ostracized and compromised by having what is for most people a simple skin infection no worse than a moderate case of eczema. Accept that you have herpes and that you'll likely have it for the rest of your life and understand that having herpes doesn't make you less moral, less ethical, less attractive, less worthy in any way than before you became infected.

3. Get out of the closet. Most of the stigma around herpes is self-imposed by those of us - including myself who have herpes. Tell your close friends and family members that you have herpes. Reach out for support and understanding the same way you would if you had a non-sexually transmitted disease. Most often the way others will react to you is a reflection of how you feel about and project yourself. The more you are at peace with your herpes the more likely it will be that you will find support and understanding in the community around you. Sixty percent of the adult population has herpes 1 or 2 so you are a member of the majority not some obscure minority.

4. Make Peace with the virus. Stress and conflict are major triggers for outbreaks. At this time there is no cure for herpes and viruses have shown themselves to be resourceful organisms well equipped for survival. I'm not suggesting that you rejoice at having this organism take up residence in your body, but the reality is that we are hosts for billions of organisms. My suggestion is to make peace with the herpes virus rather than waging war on it. Find your own way of co-existing with it in a manner which does not stimulate outbreaks and allows you to live as symptom free as possible. Hypnosis, Self-hypnosis, Creative Visualization or simply speaking to the virus may accomplish this. Please note that it has been clinically proven that people who use self-hypnosis experience 50% fewer outbreaks than those who do not.

Listen to your Natropractica Self-Hynosis CDs at least once per week if in outbreak mode- if you do not have the cds please do order them. They can be ordered from http://www.herpesbook.com or you can email me directly.

I commissioned hypnotherapist Karen Miller to create a self-hypnosis programme based on this book to give my readers and patients another tool to help them with the often challenging process of making peace with herpes.

This simple, effective self-hypnosis programme will help you stop having outbreaks, help you deal with stress and other triggers for outbreaks, help you sleep better at night, and most importantly will help ease the guilt, shame and anger often experienced by those with herpes.

The self-hypnosis CDs expand on all the themes in the book and will become a welcome part of your routine.

Here are a few words from Karen Miller on the hypnosis CDs:

Hello, my name is Karen Miller. I'm a hypnotherapist and I've designed this series of recordings to accompany Christopher Scipio's book, Making Peace with Herpes. By using these recordings you can learn to bring yourself into a deep state of hypnosis. This will facilitate your well being by allowing you to profoundly relax, to release stress and to feel good about yourself, to tap into your body's extensive capacity for wellness and to learn to alleviate discomfort. Further it can help you to integrate the core message of Christopher's work and truly come into a state of peace and deep healing.

To begin, I'd like to talk with you about what hypnosis is. For those of you who have never been in hypnosis you may have no notion of what it might feel like. Or you may have seen a stage show hypnotist working and may wonder how those techniques could possibly be useful to you. So let me explain what you can expect:

Hypnosis is a naturally occurring state that practically all humans can access. Just as we can all sleep and we can all become engrossed in a good book, we can all enter a state of hypnosis.

It is and it feels very normal.

Have you ever driven your car and been busy thinking about the events of your day? So busy thinking that in fact you found yourself all the way home in your driveway with no recollection of when or how you made that left turn through the busy intersection a few blocks back?

That's an example of a very commonly experienced trance state. And that's precisely what hypnosis feels like. Your awareness is heightened and focused and that focus allows you to achieve some remarkable things.

You will relax, you will visualize, feel or imagine experiences to support your goals and you will be able to absorb positive suggestions in a very effective way. Hypnosis works, in part, because for lots of states of consciousness the brain can't discern between an event vividly imagined and the real event. Exactly the same things are happening in exactly the same parts of the brain.

You will be present, you will be in control and you will feel remarkable. You can go into as light or as deep a state as you like and you will get better and better at entering that state each time you listen to any of the tracks on this recording. Begin by listening to the tracks in the Daily Tools for Well-Being section. These form the core of this program and you can listen to them as often as you would like. If you are experiencing any diffculty staying motivated to do those things which you know would be to your benefit and that would facitliate your healing, then be sure to listen to the Fork in the Road track to increase your motivation. Finally, I hope you will also take the time to work through the tracks in the Deep Release Section. That section contains some of the most effective methods of creating profound change that I know of. It has been my wish and my intent in creating this program to share with you the methods of healing that have worked so well for my clients. Enjoy them and enjoy coming into your balance. I wish you very well indeed!

5. Respect Your body. No matter what substances or

strategies you use to manage the disease, you still need a healthy immune system and good overall health to achieve optimum results. Treat your whole person. Respect your body. I recommend strongly that you refrain from smoking, drinking coffee, alcohol abuse, drug abuse, and any manner of behaviour you know to be physically or emotionally self-destructive. I highly recommend Yoga, Tai Chi and Qi-Gong as daily practices that will help balance your body and mind and contribute greatly to your ability to deal with the disease. Please take up one of more of these practices if you haven't already done so. I also recommend you also consider taking a martial arts class.

A Guided Daily Visualization Exercise for Herpes

You are in a temple. You are feeling warm, like a buoyant being held up by water. The weight of the world is off your shoulders.

You are at absolute peace yet you remain alert and curious. Beyond you is a stone staircase leading downwards. You step up to the precipice and begin to climb downwards.

You are seeking out the herpes virus. You have neither the spirit of confrontation or anger with you. You are seeking the virus with curiosity and openness.

With each stair you descend you are becoming even more relaxed and grounded.

You descend lower and lower into the depths of the wondrous

temple.

You feel warm water at your feet and you climb down lower and lower into the water. The water feels like home to you. This all feels like home.

You are now completely submerged in the water and you breathe effortlessly and deeply.

You reach the bottom of the staircase and you see a red glowing light ahead. You walk towards this light.

You reach the light which is a crimson red and you understand that this is the herpes virus. Your herpes virus.

You feel the virus regarding you with the same curiosity and anticipation that is in you. You step into the virus' red glowing light and you can now feel the spirit of the virus.

You are now connected with the herpes virus, it understands you and you understand it. There is no fear or resentment or anger, just understanding and peace.

You acknowledge to the virus that it has been on earth far longer than human beings and has it's own unique place in the universe. You acknowledge that the virus is not your enemy and that you have no choice but to make a peaceful co-existence together since you will the sharing the same body for life.

The virus thanks you for having the humility to make the journey and to come with the spirit of peace and understanding. The virus and you agree that the virus will stay dormant as long as you stay in equilibrium. You acknowledge that if you fall out of balance the virus will re-activate. The virus agrees to not seek to infect others through you as long as you stay in equilibrium.

You step away from the virus knowing that the peace agreement is fully understood.

You see and feel that the virus' crimson red glow is now changing; the colour is now muting as is the luminescence. You watch with curiosity and the virus fades to a dark, gray, dim light.

You understand that the virus is now dormant and is already keeping its part of the new understanding. You vow to yourself to treat your body as a temple and to stay in balance with your diet, emotions and lifestyle.

You now feel a new and profound connection with all of nature, understanding that viruses and other microorganisms are the dominant force on this planet and you have now learned to live in harmony with your herpes virus.

You begin to climb up the staircase of the temple.

You emerge from the water feeling younger, lighter and happier.

You climb to the top of the temple and open your eyes. You see a whole new day a whole new way.

My Natropractica Remedies
(This section is information only relevant to those who wish to take my herpes remedies)

Your long-term management of your herpes is divided into two phases: Outbreak Mode and Non-Outbreak Mode.

Outbreak Mode:
Consider yourself in Outbreak Mode if you have not gone at least 60-90 days without symptoms. Symptoms include sores, rashes, fissures, or any unusual eruptions on your skin as well as any itching, tingling, burning, pain or numbness. Just because there are no sores doesn't mean you're not having outbreaks. During Outbreak Mode, you are required to email me weekly to describe your emotional, mental and physical health. If you cannot or will not do this let me know.

When you are still in outbreak mode I expect you to follow the protocol to the letter. Nobody is perfect and there may be slips here and there, but if you cannot commit to following the protocol to the letter, especially in doing yoga 20 minutes per day, 7 days a week and abstaining from caffeine and nuts and if you are a woman- inserting the antiviral gel daily in your vagina at bedtime (if you have herpes below the waist), please do not start my protocol.

While you are in outbreak mode we will also be having a monthly follow-up phone consultation.

Non-Outbreak Mode:
When you have gone at least 60-90 days without symptoms you are in non-outbreak mode. Which means you no longer have to take the remedies I make for you daily, but will just keep a set on hand in case symptoms arise in the future. It also means that you need only email me once per month to update me on your health- you can write more often if you like.

In non-outbreak mode you are free to re-introduce nuts and/or caffeine into your diet, one thing at a time, to see if your immune system can tolerate it. If you get an outbreak, you'll know that your body cannot handle the offending substance.

123

In non-outbreak mode you are still required to insert the antiviral gel daily if you are a woman, and are still strongly encouraged to continue the yoga routine and taking the recommended supplements.

If you are a woman aged 35-55, in non-outbreak mode and having symptoms of a hormone imbalance, I strongly encourage you to get a bio-identical progesterone cream from your pharmacy until you are finished menopause or ask me to help you with hormone balancing herbs, to make sure your hormones are well-balanced because hormone imbalances can bring on a return of outbreaks and will worsen your herpes as your hormones get further out of balance.

Once we have stabilized your herpes, feel free to ask for my help with any other health issues that may come up even if it's as common as a cold or as vexing as vulvodynia, insomnia, digestive issues or anything else. Even though I am a viral specialist, I have a large herbal dispensary and can treat any problem you have that doesn't require surgery or a trip to the emergency room.

Whether or not you are in outbreak mode it's vitally important that you get 7-8.5 hours of sleep each day. If you cannot get that much sleep it's

imperative that you make it up with either naps or extra sleep on your days off. As few as four days in a row of less than 7 hours of sleep can cause an outbreak and weaken your immune system.

It is vitally important that you take the remedies daily while still in outbreak mode. 6-12 months of daily immune support is usually the time your body needs stop having regular outbreaks- but no two people get herpes the same way, so your time frame may be shorter or longer, but there are no short-cuts or magical quick-fixes in treating herpes holistically.

If you miss a dose please double up on the next dose. It's better to take the does at the same approximate time each day. If you have a busy schedule you can make a whole days worth of remedy and take it with you..

If you cannot or will not commit to taking the remedies daily for a minimum of six months please do not even begin the protocol because it's counter-productive for us to waste your money or my time and remedies if you are not willing to make a minimum commitment to the protocol.

Internal Use:

The remedies are strong herbal medicine and may not taste good. It's best to boil the powder on low heat in a covered pan for 10-20 minutes, you can use less than 1/2 cup of water if you like. It's best to swallow both herb and water. If away from home you can simply add hot water to the powder and prepare this way.

It's best to take the dose at least 1 hour after and one hour before meals.

Daily: On days without symptoms take the immune formula as directed on the label. If you are a woman, use the antiviral gel during sex but also insert a small amount of the antiviral gel in your vagina at bedtime every night. Store the gel in the fridge when not in use. If you get your herpes above the waist you can apply the gel topically to your lips or other area one or more times per day.

During an Outbreak: Take your recommended dose every two to four hours on onset of prodromal symptoms (itching, tingling, burning,) during waking hours during first 24 hours. Then every 4 to 6 hours during waking hours until Symptoms disappear.

Topical Use:

There's nothing more effective to apply to a herpes sore than a black tea bag- organic preferred, that has been steeped in hot water for an hour or more. Apply the wet tea bag often to your sores and you can also tear the bag slightly to expose the tea leaves directly to your skin. Unless directed otherwise you can also apply the Immune formula with your fingers or q-tip or cotton ball to the area of lesions or the area where lesions appear every 30 to

60 minutes during waking hours for the first 24 hours of symptoms (this refers to the prodrome, it's important to start applying the liquid even before lesions appear). After the first 24 hours apply the liquid as often as needed until lesions crust over and/or symptoms disappear, every 4-6 hours is the minimum but you can apply more often if you choose.

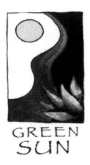

GREEN
SUN

Holistically Healing Herpes

A life-long herpes infection can affect every aspect of your life. The physical symptoms are obvious but herpes is usually a far more devastating disease emotionally, mentally and socially than it ever is physically. Since herpes can affect your whole life you need to make changes to your whole life in order to have the greatest success in living a herpes-free reality. This is what holistic healing is. In holistic medicine healing the whole person is the goal. With herpes you need to heal the way you think about herpes, the way you feel about having herpes. You need to heal how you perceive your place in the community as a person with herpes; you need to heal your love-life and your sex-life as a person with herpes. Merely popping a pill does not address any of this. This is the failure of synthetic impersonal medicine. Medicine without humanity, compassion and understanding is not medicine at all. Medicine that does not take the time to treat you as an individual and address the many levels on which a disease affects a person is not medicine at all.

• Avoid L-lysine. Long-term use of L-lysine can actually impair your immune system. Get your lysine from your diet rather than a pill.

• Avoid magical quick-fixes for herpes such as D.M.S.O and hydrogen peroxide, nonoxydol-9, BHT, MMS, etc. There are no quick-fixes for herpes.

Chapter 14:

Self-Empowerment: Further Steps to Greater Holistic Health

For any suggestion I make to you to have any chance of resonating with you it would have to be simple and make good common sense. Following the protocol outlined in the previous section is all one has to do to manage herpes holistically, but if you wish to take your holistic health to an even higher level the following steps are both simple and practical and also have the additional benefit of being proven effective over a long period of time. Read with an open mind and you just may find yourself healthier and happier in ways beyond your expectations.

Drink Natural Water.

My colleague and master herbalist Katherine Nelson in

Vancouver, Canada taught me about the importance of drinking natural spring water. Proper hydration is the most important element of healthy nutrition. If you are drinking distilled water or filtered water you are drinking de-mineralized water, which contain no electrolytes and cannot properly hydrate you. Nature provides us with natural water; the key to life on this planet. Hydrate yourself with natural unfiltered spring water.

Eat Hemp Seeds.

Much has been discovered and written recently about the importance of essential fatty acids. Hemp seeds not only have the highest amount of omega 3 and 6 found in nature but hemp is full of amino acids and is 30% protein. The protein in hemp seeds is the closest to the protein in your own body and the easiest to digest. Four tablespoons of hemp seeds every morning will provide you with energy and vitality for the whole day and help you avoid the mid-afternoon low blood sugar slump. Sorry to disappoint the stoners out there but the hemp seeds in your health food store contain no THC and are completely legal. Hemp seeds also taste way better than flax and can be nicely placed on yoghurt, in smoothies, on salads, eaten straight, baked into cookies and brownies and anything else your heart may desire.

Drink Apple Cider Vinegar.

Do yourself and your body the greatest favour by drinking a two teaspoons of organic apple cider vinegar a day- (you can dilute it in water or juice). It will help clear phlegm and mucous from your body, help protect you from colds and sinus infections, protect your veins and arteries from plaque buildup and keep your whole body well-tuned.

Drink Aloe Vera Juice.

Since the time of the Egyptians, aloe vera juice has been one of the most universally used medicines on the planet. Aloe vera juice coats and protects your stomach and is a great digestive tonic. It is anti-inflammatory and helpful for IBS, ulcers, and arthritis. Aloe vera juice lowers blood pressure, helps to balance blood sugar, boosts the immune system and may even be helpful for cancer. I recommend two ounces per day in water or juice.

Grow and Drink Lemon Balm Tea.

Lemon balm is my second favourite plant. It is a green Goddess. She is a wonder nervine to help relax your nerves and avoid triggering an outbreak. She is also a wonderful antiviral. Lemon balm grows everywhere, smells wonderful and makes one of the most delicious teas. Grow lemon balm and drink it fresh daily because dried lemon balm is too weak to be of any real use to people with herpes.

Eat Avocadoes

Avocadoes are something I recommend you eat often. It's well worth spending the extra money to get organic avocadoes. Avocadoes are an almost perfect food, they help lower bad cholesterol and lower blood pressure, they give your immune system the essential fatty acids it needs, they inhibit prostrate cancer and help your body absorbs nutrients from vegetables better.

Eat Seaweeds

Many of you may have heard about the benefits of red marine

algae for herpes and other viral illnesses. What isn't being said is that there are more than 3000 species of medicinal red marine algae in the world, with only about 20 or so being clinically shown to be effective against the Epstein Barr and herpes viruses. Most of what is sold as red marine algae in capsules is actually cheap Gigartina and other species from the Philippines and other third world countries which may have little effectiveness with herpes and which may not be harvested from clean waters. If you live near unpolluted water on either the Atlantic or Pacific coasts I encourage you to learn about and gather any local red or purple seaweeds and tincture them. In addition I encourage anyone who has herpes to eat Wakame and Dulse seaweeds from your health food store. Seaweeds contain virtually all the minerals and trace elements needed by your body. Leave the dubious red marine algae sold on the net or in the stores on the shelves.

Eat/Drink Blueberries

Blueberries are probably the best thing you could put in your body except for water. It's list of health benefits are so long that I encourage you to do a search and discover them more in depth. Some of the benefits include: anti-oxidant and anti-inflammatory, protector of brain cells, improving memory, lowers the risk of cancer, promotes urinary tract health, good for arthritis and gout, and is anti-aging.

Eat Bitter Melons

This tropical fruit looks like a light green cucumber with a bad case of acne. It can be found in any Chinatown. It has been shown to inhibit HIV and herpes and is a great all around natural anti-viral. It has also been used to treat cancer and diabetes. I encourage you to cook some bitter melon in a

Chinese stir-fry or as a side dish to any meal. Best to slice it thin and then fry with seaweed flakes or a tiny amount of sea salt. It tastes a bit bitter but no more bitter than beer, and it's great for anyone with herpes.

Eat/Drink Pomegranates

The tannins in pomegranates have been shown to be anti-viral against herpes. It is also a great natural anti-biotic and a wonderful anti-oxidant, better than green tea, certainly better than chocolate. It's a reliable cure for diarrhea. Pomegranates should be avoided if you are pregnant or breast-feeding.

Use Honey

If you have herpes honey should be the only sweetener that you use. It's superior to maple syrup or cane juice. It has strong antiviral properties, it's a good source of antioxidants, it may be helpful for ulcers, it helps reduce fatigue and dehydration and if you eat local raw honey it will help you with seasonal allergies.

Drink Dandelion Juice

In the springtime gather and juice all the above-ground parts of the dandelion, of course make sure you collect somewhere free of chemical sprays and pollution. Dandelion juice is a potent anti-herpes medicine but it also a great natural multivitamin.

Juice Grapes in your juicer.
Grapes and red wine have been long known to be helpful for herpes. What isn't commonly known is that pasteurized grape juice sold in bottles is useless for herpes because it has been

heated. If you want to use the amazing powers of the grape to help your herpes, juice the darkest grapes you can in a juicer and then strain it if it has seeds. Drinking half a cup of grape juice regularly will help anyone with herpes a great deal and will provide many other health benefits as well.

Eat Shitake Mushrooms.

The queen of the mushroom world is a great ally to anyone with herpes or without herpes. Shitake is a magnificent immune builder and is a preventative for many kinds of cancer. Shitake helps fight fatigue and stress, are rich in protein, have all the essential amino acids just like meat, milk and eggs do with far fewer calories. They also taste wonderful. Please also help stop the misinformation being put out there about medicinal mushrooms. Medicinal mushrooms unlike the common white or brown culinary mushrooms do not cause any Candida, yeast or fungal problems. Mushrooms and Seaweeds are the oldest plants in the world and are a great addition to anyone's health.

Beyond Herpes:

An African Bush Doctor's Prescription for Greater Holistic Health

Bush Medicine is traditional herbal medicine, the oldest system of healing in the world. Bush medicine started in Africa about 30,000 years ago. In the African-Caribbean culture, plants are referred to as "Bush" such as "fever bush" or "toothache bush" and are revered for their healing and spiritual properties. Every culture in the world practiced and still practices bush medicine to treat the physical, emotional, mental and spiritual problems of the people. Today 70% of the world's population still uses traditional herbal medicine (bush medicine) as their primary source of health care.

For the past 75 years medical doctors and drug companies have tried to discredit traditional herbal medicine, while at the same time sending ethnobotanists all around the world to acquire the knowledge of local plants from bush doctors in order to make new pharmaceutical drugs.

Often once a drug company has appropriated local plant knowledge, usually without compensating the locals in any way, they patent the plants and pressure the governments into banning the local population from having access to the plants they have depended on for millennia. Fortunately there is now a worldwide effort underway to protect local plant knowledge from unethical exploitation. People are returning to their traditional herbalists because of the failure of pharmaceutical drugs to treat chronic health problems safely and effectively. I am from a long-line of African bush doctors. My family has practiced traditional herbal medicine for ten generations. My grandmother was a prominent bush doctor in Trinidad, the country of my birth. The African-Caribbean culture is a largely intact culture where we have retained much of the knowledge of our bush doctors. Here are some simple tips for improving your health from me, Christopher Scipio, your friendly, neighbourhood bush doctor.

1. Eat less. Unless you are very physically active you are probably eating a third more calories than you need. Excessive caloric intake is one of the biggest factors in reducing life expectancy.

2. Don't eat alone. People eat too quickly, chew their food less, and tend to consume less nutritional meals when they are eating alone. Having company provides many health benefits and is much better for your mental and emotional well-being.

2A. Pay attention to your eating environment. Loud noises, lack of a comfortable sitting position, too many distractions and a less than peaceful environment can all contribute to digestive problems and may cascade into other health issues. Eating in a relaxed quiet environment with good company is a great habit to get into.

3. Along the theme of eating less, **use smaller plates and cutlery** and consider using chop sticks or your fingers to eat with. The oversized cutlery just promotes the wolfing down of food. I love using chopsticks for lots of different kinds of meals and there is much sensual pleasure with eating with your fingers the way Africans do.

4. Reduce your carbs, especially bread and pasta. Obesity and many of the health problems that go with it like diabetes were virtually unknown until we started consuming such large quantities of bread, pasta and baked goods. I recommend not eating bread or pasta more than three or four times per week and substituting beans and dishes like hummus as a replacement.

5. Get and use a juicer. The juice you buy in a store is dead. Many juice enzymes die within an hour of extraction. Most juices have been pasteurized to further deplete their nutritional value. Making your own juice is a joy. I like starting the day with a blend of carrot, apple, Hawaiian ginger and beet juice, but there are so many juices to discover. I recommend the book on healing juices by Heinermann.

6. Cook your own food. It is more than worth the time. I know you are busy but you can work cooking into any schedule. Consider getting a slow cooker. Consider cooking large batches on your days off and keeping them ready in the freezer. Cooking your own food is the only way of knowing what actually is put into your food, plus it sends the right message to your body that you care.

6A. Don't assume restaurant food is healthy. Many restaurants are fond of using iceberg lettuce which is very cheap and is usually grown in high-tech hydroponic factories but has virtually no nutritional value and don't even ask about the chemicals used to keep lettuce looking "fresh". Most restaurants don't use organic ingredients and many restaurants use microwaves to heat their meals. Just take a tour of the kitchen of your favourite restaurants and you may be horrified.

7. Bless your food and remember where it comes from.
This modern life is a very disconnected from reality kind of life. Often there is little thought given to where food comes from, how it was harvested and processed and by whom. Do you know where you food came from? If not you better bless it and bless it well before you take it and all the vibes that go along with it into your sensitive body.

8. Balance yourself daily with Yoga, Tai-chi or Qi- Gong.
Twenty minutes a day in your own home of one of these practices and I'll personally guarantee your health will improve no matter how healthy you were beforehand. You can go to classes as well but what I recommend is that you empower yourself by learning how to do simple routines at home so you are not dependant on a class.

9. Get and give a massage at least once per month. Weekly is even better. Give and receive this vital practice as often as possible. Even a mediocre massage is better than none at all so recruit your partner or a friend if you cannot access a professional and don't be reluctant to lay your hands on others as well.

10. Have more sex. Marvin G. knew what he was talking about when he sang "Sexual Healing". If you can work it into your moral parameters to have more sex, do. A regular orgasm is a great prescription. Please do practice safer sex and consider using an anti-viral gel.

11. Don't forget to laugh. Laughter is great medicine. Give yourself permission to be silly, don't be so serious and you'll have a longer and happy life.

12. Just say no to drugs. Ronald and Nancy Regan were worried about recreational drugs and I agree that recreational drugs are harmful to your health, but the drugs that I see devastating the community's health the most are coffee, alcohol and cigarettes, in that order. Don't believe the self-serving propaganda from the Starbucks lobby about the possible benefits of drinking coffee. There are no net benefits to drinking coffee and it is particularly devastating to women's health as is heavy alcohol consumption and cigarettes.

13. Eat like an adult not a child. You are a big boy/girl now so eat like one. Don't be a slave to cravings and food addictions. Eat for nutritional value and not strictly for taste or as an emotional panacea. On my hot list of non-nutritional foods are chocolate, ice cream, sodas, white bread, white rice, and white pasta.

14. Eat soft foods. Eat wet foods. Softer foods are much easier for your body to digest and are much more likely to have a high water content. Wet foods are also easier to digest and help provide the water you need. Your body is mostly water, the earth is mostly water, so try to limit dry, hard, dead foods like crackers, bread, and cereals and embrace soft wet foods like soups, purees (I love baba ganoush), fruit, steamed vegetables, smoothies, organic plain yoghurt, etc.

The human body is a wondrous miracle of engineering and grace. Treat your body well and it will reward you with many years of health and happiness. Neglect or abuse your body at your own peril.

Christopher Scipio
Herbalist
Holistic Viral Specialist
African Bush Doctor

The Future of Herpes

Without a cure for herpes likely in our lifetime, I feel passionate about creating a much better climate for those who will get herpes in the future, especially the pre-teens, teenagers and college-age students who are the majority of new herpes cases currently.

Herpes education is a cause worth getting involved with. I realize that everyone has different interests and inclinations, not everyone is going to want to be publicly identified with herpes. Until someone is brave enough and cares enough to start a herpes charity it's up to all of us as individuals to try and make a difference in our communities. The old saying that "if you are not part of the solution you are part of the problem" has never been truer than it is of herpes today.

You are an important and influential member of your community whether you realize it or not. You can and do influence the people around you, even if it's subtle, even if it's unconscious.

If you choose to stay in the herpes closet and be ashamed then not only are you enslaving yourself but you are denying other people the chance to be positively influenced by you. Make peace with your own herpes and practice safer responsible sexuality and share those experiences with those you feel comfortable sharing it with, even if it's only your friends and family. Six out of every ten people you know has herpes whether they admit it or not, whether they know it or not.

The AIDS epidemic only got under control because of courageous people speaking out like Magic Johnson, Ryan White, Elizabeth Taylor, Madonna, Greg Louganis and many others and because of the tireless and brilliant work by organizations such as the Gay Men's Health Crisis. They got the word out about holistic HIV treatment and HIV prevention.

Sadly not one celebrity admits to having herpes and there are no national spoke-persons talking about it prominently in the media. You don't hear about it on Oprah, you don't hear about it anywhere.

It's up to all of us with herpes to reach and teach others. There's so much bad information out there and people trying to take advantage of our collective desperation.

For those of you like me who are more bold, go to your local radio and television stations and print media and talk about herpes prevention and holistic treatment. Don't leave people out there thinking that expensive drug therapy is their only option. Discuss safer sexuality especially to the 13-22 year olds. Write your blogs, make art about herpes, write songs, make t-shirts, join or start internet message boards, make podcasts, become holistic herpes treatment specialists, do whatever the spirit moves you to do, but don't ever feel that you are powerless to make a difference.

It's imperative that we build up our immune systems and practice safer sex for another important reason: Herpes and HIV aren't going to be the last pandemics from the world of microorganisms. It has been predicted by many holistic healers and scientists that within our lifetime there will be at least one or two sexually transmitted viruses or bacteria that will be far worse than herpes or HIV. Having herpes is a gateway on your skin that allows any other sexually transmitted virus or microbe to penetrate into your body.

So those who do not treat and protect themselves will be the hardest hit by any future diseases. Many of the people currently infected with HIV and HPV had herpes first.

Feel free at any time to email me with questions, comments observations, herbs to try, anything at all. I love being a part of the herpes nation. You can also ask to recive our free monthly newsletter full of health tips, stories from our readers with herpes on how they are overcoming the disease, healthy recipes and more.

How To Get This Book For Free?

*If after reading this book you're interested in having a phone consultation to ask questions, get support and advice or wish to start my holistic herpes treatment programme- I will deduct the price of this book from the cost of your phone consultation. Please either write to me directy at **christopher.scipio@gmail. com** or book your consultation through my site at **http://www.natropractica.com***

If you have enjoyed reading this book and wish to enhance your natural herpes management plan even more, I strongly encourage you to get the self-hypnosis CDs that are designed to work with this book.

For more information on my antiviral gel to make safer sex even safer go to http://www.antiviralgel.com

Nine Ways

The Universe is the Great Healer, Nature the Great Doctor

Our Bodies are the Great Temples

To Heal is to Love, to Love is to Heal

We are All Great Lovers; We are All Great Healers, if We Choose to Be

Healing is Simple, Natural and Pleasurable. Healing is Beyond Substance, Beyond Ego, Beyond Definition- Healing is Magic

Medicine surrounds US Everywhere; Plant, Animal, Mineral and Energetic

Cultural Disorder (Being Out of Synch with Nature) is the Great Disease

Beholding The Natural World with Sincerity, Wonder and Humility is the Way to See the Medicine and Healing Miracles All Around Us.

Any Human Being Unmoved by the Beauty and Miraculousness of Nature is Beyond the Reach of Natural Healing.

68203088R00081

Made in the USA
Lexington, KY
05 October 2017